Economic Benefits of Enhanced Fitness

Roy J. Shephard, MD, PhD
University of Toronto

Human Kinetics Publishers, Inc.
Champaign, Illinois

Library of Congress Cataloging-in-Publication Data

Shephard, Roy J.
  Economic benefits of enhanced fitness.

  Bibliography: p.
  Includes index.
  1. Physical fitness—Economic aspects—Canada.
2. Labor and laboring classes—Canada—Physical
training—Costs. 3. Physical fitness—Economic aspects.
4. Labor and laboring classes—Physical training.
I. Title.
GV510.C2S54 1986   613.7'0971   86-410
ISBN 0-87322-060-9

Developmental Editor: Sue Wilmoth, PhD
Production Director: Ernest Noa
Copy Editor: Kristen LaDuke-Gallup
Typesetter: Sandra Meier
Text Design: Julie Szamocki
Text Layout: Lezli Harris
Cover Design: Jack Davis
Printed By: Braun-Brumfield, Inc.

ISBN: 0-87322-060-9

Printed in the United States of America

10 9 8 7 6 5 4 3 2 1

Human Kinetics Publishers, Inc.
Box 5076, Champaign, IL 61820

Contents

Acknowledgments

As in my other writings, I owe much to a number of generous colleagues. Blake Ferris and Sandy Keir of Fitness and Amateur Sport, Ottawa; Burt Perrin of Fitness Ontario; and Russ Kisby of ParticipACTION have all contributed freely of their ideas and resources, while Rob Beamish, Alan Detsky, John Howard, and Reiner Jaakson have each offered kind and constructive criticism after reading the original manuscript. To all of these individuals and others who have helped my task in various ways I express warmest thanks while recognizing my responsibility for errors that may have crept back into the final version of the text. I also much appreciate the generous financial support of the Fitness and Amateur Sport branch of the Canadian Government, which has sustained both the conduct of background research and the preparation of the manuscript.

Roy J. Shephard

Preface

*Aggregate leisure spending is an area of research that appears to have
been almost entirely neglected by academic and government researchers.*
(Martin & Mason, 1983, p. 9)

The internationally acclaimed *A new perspective on the health of Canadians* (Lalonde, 1974) did much to reshape medical priorities not only in Canada but also in other parts of the world. It focused attention upon the value of prevention in several major health fields, including the promotion of physical activity. A decade later, the ever-increasing costs of conventional medical technology, the insistence of an aging population upon expensive secondary and tertiary care, and a shrinking tax base are forcing further examination of both the costs and the benefits of a strategy built around preventive medicine and the fostering of a healthy lifestyle.

Cost-benefit and cost-effectiveness analyses are increasingly applied in the approval or rejection of policy options by university administrators, corporation executives, and senior civil servants in various levels of government. Rather than distributing available funds by instinct, hunches, or the "old-boy network," fiscal decisions are being made in rational, carefully analyzed, and defensible terms.

To many who have been major recipients of the public purse, this development is greatly feared. Anxiety is particularly acute where an option is of dubious merit. While flattery, manipulation, and the art of Machiavelli may have yielded funds in the past, economic analyses are resistant to such blandishments. The physical educator and fitness enthusiast should nevertheless welcome this modern approach, since analyses to date suggest quite favorable cost/benefit and cost-effectiveness ratios for exercise.

In a report to the Council of Europe, Rodgers (1978) stressed that the level of sports finance was a key factor affecting participation in sport. He thus urged the council to make "much more serious attempts to discover the total level of sports spending, public and private, and its structure down the hierarchy of administrative units."

The value of funding new fitness initiatives has been strongly encouraged by several recent developments, including (a) the epidemiological work of Paffenbarger (1977) and Morris et al. (1973), which suggests that vigorous physical activity has a strong association with protection against cardiac disease; (b) the Toronto Life Assurance study (Shephard, 1984), which has shown that employee fitness programs not only improve individual fitness, but also reduce industrial absenteeism, employee turnover, costs of medical care, and appraised age (as assessed from the Health Hazard Appraisal inventory); (c) calculations suggesting that an enhancement of physical activity among the elderly might reduce their demands for institutional care (Shephard, 1978); and (d) the potential of labor-intensive recreation to both satisfy the demand for new jobs and fill the increased free time of the late 1980s.

Nevertheless, the physical educator must learn the basic language of the economist if these inherently persuasive arguments are to be presented in terms that the modern executive will understand and accept. Such a vocabulary and an understanding are needed equally by the young investigator, penning a first grant proposal in fitness and health; the corporate fitness supervisor, wishing an extension of noon-hour exercise classes; the municipal recreation coordinator, advocating construction of a new swimming pool; and the executive of a health promotion agency competing for public funding against other apparently worthy causes.

The present book is intended to meet this need. For the first time, it draws together information on the fiscal benefits of increased physical activity and presents this material at a level appropriate for the professional who wishes to evaluate and justify the programs in which he or she is involved. Examples are selected from the entire field of fitness and active recreation. New information is presented that suggests very favorable cost-benefit ratios for several aspects of fitness programing, with respect to both health status and the industrial economy. A physically active lifestyle is shown to have more than intrinsic merit. It is also a key first step toward the initiation of change in several of the other health fields examined by LaFramboise (1973), Lalonde (1974), and R. Morgan (1977). A comprehensive analysis of costs and benefits demonstrates the social and fiscal desirability of increased expenditures in the field of fitness promotion. At the same time, it brings to light gaps in our understanding of the economics of fitness and health. Accordingly, specific research is recommended to fill these gaps in current knowledge.

Reports from our laboratory and elsewhere have suggested that a number of important social and economic benefits are associated with an increase of physical activity. Gains are seen in the workplace (greater productivity and reduced absenteeism, turnover, and industrial injuries), in the health-care system (fewer physician visits and less need for hospital utilization and geriatric care), and in lifestyle (reduction of appraised age and a lesser incidence of cigarette and alcohol abuse). Each of the "western" nations might save billions of dollars if regular exercise were to be adopted by their entire populations. Nevertheless, a detailed analysis is needed to assess whether all classes of subjects benefit equally and also to determine possible overlap among various categories of postulated benefits.

The text thus looks at both monetary and nonmonetary costs and benefits of enhanced physical activity in relation to personal, sociocultural, industrial, environmental, and geriatric sectors of the economy. Personal aspects include commitments of time (as a participant or volunteer leader) and the impact of regular exercise upon physical and psychological health, medical and rehabilitation costs, nutrition, lifestyle, drug abuse, and education. Sociocultural considerations include the importance of physical activity relative to other social priorities, the impact of fitness promotion upon the economic sectors of tourism, spectator sports, consumer entertainment, beer and cigarette manufacturing, and the influence of disposable income upon overall leisure behavior.

Physical activity is next discussed in the context of automation. Emphasis is put upon the potential of the fitness market to create jobs, both directly (through labor-intensive professional services) and indirectly (through the production of specialized equipment and clothing), while sustaining the life-satisfaction of those who are unemployed. Detailed statistics are also presented on the industrial benefits of physical activity such as enhanced productivity, reduced absenteeism, lower employee turnover, and less frequent occupational injuries. The possible contribution of enhanced activity to the reduction of geriatric costs is then explored.

The various types of active leisure are assessed critically, in terms of both their dollar costs and the impact of the necessary facilities upon the environment. A final chapter looks at ethical issues, in particular, the promotion of lifestyle and personal responsibility versus corporate, societal change. Gaps in knowledge are discussed, with recommendations concerning further data collection, and an interim balance sheet is developed to show the likely costs and benefits of physical fitness promotion in a modern industrial society.

Topics not explored in any detail include (a) the impact of governmental initiatives upon the response of private delivery agencies and (b) the impact of elitist or specialist programing upon the more general fitness of the community. Unfortunately, accurate statistics are lacking on these two issues.

However, an extensive bibliography gives access to other recent papers that have a bearing upon the economics of fitness promotion and delivery.

chapter 1

Principles of Health Economics

Ideally, this article should begin with a mathematical model, an equa-tion. On the left, we should put together contributions and expenditures in terms of hours, money and effort. On the right, we should enter the profits in terms of years of life, money and quality of life. Unfortunately, it is not that easy. (Waaler & Hjort, 1982, p. 265)

The basic problem of recreation and leisure provision . . . is the lack of a coherent financial policy. (Chartered Institute of Public Financing and Accountancy, 1979, p. 1)

Economics may be defined as the science of managing expenditures. The original Greek word *oikonomia* referred to the management of a house-hold, usually by a steward, and the same was true of medieval English (*yconomie*, or *howsolde keepynge*). However, the Scottish philosopher Adam Smith, in his classical work *The Wealth of Nations* (1776), extended the con-cept to cover the art of managing the resources of a people and its govern-ment. This concept currently encompasses the entire theoretical science of the laws of production and distribution of wealth.

If wealth were limitless, the economist would not be in great demand. Unfortunately, governments, industries, and universities are all becom-ing increasingly aware of the limitations to wealth, and a corresponding burgeoning interest exists in the techniques of fiscal management.

What is the source of this apparently shrinking wealth? The three basic resources are labor, land, and capital. Labor includes both manual and mental work applied to natural resources; in many countries, an aging population and demands for more extended education are reducing the labor force (or, as gerontologists prefer to express it, the dependency ratio is increasing—see chapter 5).

"Land" was originally envisaged in an agricultural sense, but now includes all natural resources such as forests, mineral ores, and gasoline. Again, simple observation shows that all forms of land are becoming in-creasingly scarce as the world consumption of commodities grows. "Cap-ital" comprises that fraction of a worker's production that he or she does not consume; it allows an accumulation of materials and equipment that can be applied to increased productivity in the future. Wise investment in automation might—at least in the short-term—lead to a substantial increase in wealth, but at present the problem in many nations is that the laborer's surplus is directed toward the purchase of rapidly outdated military hardware, which leaves a shrinking margin for investment in such concerns as fitness and health.

Major corporations also face ever-increasing competition from developing nations that can offer cheap labor, cheap raw materials, and (often) a careless disregard for employee health and safety. The funding of universities, equally, is being reduced in response to an aging population and a popular distrust of academicians.

Thus government, business, and university administrators are increasingly applying the tools of the modern economist—cost-benefit and cost-effectiveness analyses—to evaluate the return on both new and established programs. Review is focused particularly upon so-called "social" programs, such as fitness and health, because some administrators view these items as luxurious frills that can be eliminated without cost to society. Some fitness professionals fear economic probing, but if time is taken to learn the techniques of the health economist (Office of Technology Assessment, 1980), the case for future funding of fitness and health initiatives becomes even more compelling.

Before considering possible benefits from enhanced physical activity and the promotion of physical fitness, we will thus take a brief look at the language and tools of the economist, beginning with a short glossary of common economic terms defined in the context of this monograph.

Glossary of Economic Terms

Capital—the unconsumed surplus product of labor working on land, as defined.

Cardinal System of Evaluation—approval of a program reaching an arbitrary cost-benefit or cost-effectiveness ratio.

Compensating Variation—the willingness of the consumer to make good the shortfall in external funding for a program.

Consumer Price Index (CPI)—the cost of a standard "basket" of goods and services, expressed as a percentage of their cost in a criterion year (e.g., 1971 = 100).

Cost-Benefit Ratio—an analysis based upon the ratio of the dollar costs of a program to an assessment of benefits, also made in dollar terms.

Cost-Effectiveness Ratio—an analysis based upon the ratio of the dollar costs of a program to an assessment of benefits, expressed in arbitrary terms (e.g., 1 year of life).

Dependency Ratio—the number of dependents (children, handicapped, and elderly) expressed as a ratio to the population of working age.

Discount Rate—an expression of society's willingness to invest capital for the benefit of future generations (often approximated as the ratio of return on long-term government bonds, or the yield on industrial investments).

Employment Rate—the proportion of adults of working age who are seeking employment and have found full-time jobs.

Equivalent Variation—the alternative investment that is needed to compensate for withdrawal of a specific program.

Exchange Rate—the rate accepted by international banks for exchange of currency on a given date (e.g., US $1.00 = CDN $1.34 February 1985).

Gross Domestic Product (GDP)—the market worth of goods, services, and domestic activity in a nation over a specific period.

Gross National Product (GNP)—the market worth of goods and services produced by a nation over a specified period.

Human Capital—investment in formal education and training.

Impact Evaluation—an analysis of a program based upon its impact on the target (e.g., recruitment of 25% of a target population).

Inflation—a decrease in the real value of a currency, commonly assessed in terms of increases in the Consumer Price Index.

Intangible Costs—intangible good or bad outcomes of a specific situation (e.g., the loss of production caused by personal grief).

Investment—direction of capital to a specific program (e.g., $4 of private capital might be attracted for the investment of $1 of government capital, thus causing a multiplier effect of 4.00 to 1.0).

Labor—the effort applied by humans to all forms of land, including both physical and mental work.

Land—all of the resources provided by nature, such as agricultural land and minerals.

Marginal Costs—the change in cost associated with a change in scale of a program.

Migration—the movement of population into or out of a country (immigration and emigration, respectively).

Multiplier Effect—see *Investment*.

Opportunity Cost—the time a person forgoes through participation in a program which might have been spent in other profitable ways commonly estimated as an average wage—e.g., $10h^{-1}).

Ordinal System—an arbitrary criterion of effectiveness, established after community discussion (e.g., an added year of life merits a $100,000 program investment).

Outcome Evaluation—analysis of a program based upon an outcome measure (e.g., a 25% reduction of ischemic heart disease in the targeted community).

Participation Rate—the proportion of the population of working age that is actively seeking work.

Price Elasticity—the change of program participation for unit change of cost.

Privatization—the transfer of responsibility for a program from government to a private entrepreneur.

Process Evaluation—analysis of an embryonic program on the basis of the process that has been established.

Producer Price Index—the price charged by producers of a group of commodities, expressed as a percentage of a criterion value (e.g., 1971 = 100).

Saturation—a point at which further investment will have little or no impact on the effectiveness of a program.

Transfer Payments—money transferred from one sector of the economy to another (e.g., taxes paid to government by an individual or a corporation).

Value—defined by most economists as the price of an article or service in dollar terms. When comparing two alternative programs or policies, a value judgment is required, and this can sometimes be facilitated by expressing the two options in cost-benefit or cost-effectiveness terms.

Wages—money paid for labor. Many cost-benefit calculations require estimates of the value of unpaid work (e.g., parenting by a spouse).

Key issues to be considered in this chapter (Drummond & Mooney, 1982) are the reasons why a program is being costed, the nature of any value decisions that must be incorporated into the analysis, problems of cost-equivalence across time and across national boundaries, accounting conventions, and the merits of cost-benefit versus cost-effectiveness analysis. Possible methods of evaluating the effectiveness of fitness promotion (process, impact, and outcome) will be addressed, and both the tactics and the strategy of fitness planning will be discussed.

Reasons for Costing

The costs of most health and fitness services vary with the context in which they are demanded. Thus we must decide why we are interested in the economics of fitness promotion. Several differing scenarios could be envisaged:

Compressing Social Services

Growing budgetary deficits might cause a government to ask, What would be the economic consequences of reducing fitness expenditures by 20%? In such a hypothetical situation, the current unit costs of fitness services and the benefits derived therefrom would be inappropriate data. The number of active individuals would probably decrease with program compression, but the residual participants would be highly committed to exercise and would persist with their habits despite deteriorating facilities and little encouragement from government.

If an employee fitness plan were to be discontinued, corporate expenditures on other forms of "welfare" programs (equivalent variation) might also be needed for a company to retain its key workers (see Mishan, 1976). Thus Morey (1983) estimated that the U.S. Navy would need to spend $3.20-$4.60 on alternative benefits for every dollar saved by a discontinuation of its fitness program. Some economists also estimate the compensating variation, or the willingness of the participant to make good the shortfall in external funding, by looking at the influence of such costs upon facility use (Sielaff, 1964). Generally, this sets a lower value upon programs than does the equivalent variation (Morey, 1983). Finally, one might inquire for which components of a program the equivalent variation exceeded the cost of the facility (Mansfield, 1971).

In general, it is unlikely that a 20% reduction of governmental fitness expenditures would help to reduce an overall economic deficit. More probably, the money would be diverted to allow a new initiative by some other arm of government to enter, and in some instances it might merely nourish "fat" in a rival program.

Reviewing Current Programs

Alternatively, government might wish to review existing programs, inquiring, What is the current cost of inducing an individual citizen to become physically active? In order to answer this question, it would be necessary to determine the minimum intensity and duration of physical activity inducing the desired benefit (such as greater health or increased productivity); subsequent steps would be to examine the percentage of the population presently achieving such a standard, the costs that are incurred thereby, and the number of citizens who would have achieved the same standard in the absence of any fitness promotion program.

A second method of assessing current programs is in terms of the investment that they stimulate. Berger (1983) distinguishes direct investment (in his example, $4.60 per $1.00 of spending by the Provincial Government), indirect spending (a multiplier effect, ranging from 1.16 for active recreation to 1.88 for associated purchases of travel, food, and accommodation), and opportunity investment by volunteers ($0.47 per $1.00). In some instances, it may be useful to distinguish the stimulation of private rather than public investment because federal and state or provincial initiatives often have their main impacts upon regional or municipal levels of government rather than upon private spending.

When evaluating disadvantaged areas of a country, examining regional multipliers is also useful (Gamble, 1975). These tend to be largest in the larger tourist regions. In the U.S., the overall regional multiplier ranges from 1.36 to 2.21, although the benefit to the personal incomes of local residents is much smaller (0.23 to 0.56). Other items to be evaluated in regional calculations are losses of local tax revenue (e.g., if a substantial acreage is allocated for park land) and the possibility that zero investment might have occurred in the absence of an initiative by central government. In this last situation, central government could legitimately claim 100% of the benefits derived from construction of a facility (Berger, 1983).

Expanding Fitness Programing

Assuming that the various cost-benefits suggested in the previous scenario appear favorable, government or industrial management might wish to expand fitness programing in order to service that 70-80% of a community or company that is currently relatively inactive. For example, Williamson and van Nieuwenhuijzen (1974) applied a simple Delphic approach to industrial absenteeism, seeking a comparison of anticipated rates between health care as presently given, optimal health care, and no health care.

When considering program expansion, account must be taken of marginal costs. Would central governmental spending continue to exert the same multiplier effect in an expanding program? Would regional interest in fitness reach the ''take-off'' point for a major private investment, or would impact upon the local tax base and entrepreneurial interest reach a point of saturation? How much increase of expenditures would be needed in order to reach and service a further 1% of a given population? Economies of scale might be possible through a fuller use of existing facilities and supervisory personnel, but the new exercise recruits would be much more costly to motivate than those who were already active (Haggerty, 1977). They would also be less likely to commit their own money and time to program participation. Price elasticity data (in the fitness context, the change of participation rates for a 1% variation in the charge per exercise session) would be very different if the base participation rate was 80% rather than 20-30%.

A further imponderable point is whether the personal and industrial benefits of physical activity would remain on a comparable scale if participation were extended to a larger segment of the population. Given that there are high absentee rates and substantial demands for physical effort on the factory floor, there might be greater relative effects upon absenteeism and productivity if fitness could be extended from its present "white-collar" base to the "blue-collar" segment of the labor force instead of expanding white-collar participation. Likewise, estimates of health-care savings need to take account of the substantial differences in the patterns of health-care demand between white- and blue-collar workers (Segall, 1981).

Developing Alternative Programing

A final reason for the costing of fitness programs might be to consider alternative approaches that would yield equivalent benefits. For example, if the focus was upon lagging productivity, it might be asked whether some type of bonus such as a longer paid holiday would induce similar gains to an employee fitness program for a smaller cost. Equally, if the concern was a rising demand for medical care, it might be thought necessary to examine the effectiveness of fitness promotion relative to a tactic such as stopping all advertising of cigarettes. In this example, it would be desirable to consider also such factors as public acceptance of legislation restricting cigarette advertising and the indirect impact of such a policy upon other aspects of the economy, particularly magazine publishing and possible alternative beneficiaries of promotional dollars.

Cost comparisons may also be required relative to more traditional forms of medical treatment. While fitness as yet lacks the well-organized antagonism that is encountered when promoting dietary change or regulation of tobacco sales (Thomas, 1979), in the long-run it could well be perceived as a threat to both the purse and the prestige of sickness-oriented medicine (Cappon, 1983).

Finally, cost comparisons may be needed among various potential fitness promotional tactics. For example, should moneys be allocated to sport or to recreation? Likewise, is it better to seek new recruits or to concentrate efforts upon improving the adherence of those already recruited (Weinstein & Stason, 1977)?

Weinstein (1983) suggested a formal basis for estimating the effectiveness, E, of alternative tactics according to the formula

$$E = \sum_{i=0}^{I-1} \sum_{j=0}^{J-1} \sum_{m=0}^{M-1} (z_{jm} \, q_{ij} \, p_i) k_i e_m$$

There are I possible values for the potency of the proposed tactic (o, $k_1, k_2 \ldots k - 1$), each assigned a corresponding prior probability (p_1 is the probability of effectiveness k_1). There are also J possible results of further experimental studies, with a probability r_j (j = 0, ... J − 1). The probability of result r_i representing the true effect K_l is then given by q_{ij} = probability $[r_j k_i]$. Finally, there are M possible changes of behavior as a result of the tactic (o, e_1 . . . . e_{M-1}), so that the probability of exposure change e_m for result r_j is Z_{jm} = probability $[e_m r_j]$.

To examine this concept in simpler and less mathematical terms, look at the effectiveness of increased physical activity in the prevention of ischemic heart disease. Current data might suggest two possible responses, k_o = 0 (no effect) or k_i = 0.5 (50% prevention of disease, established with a probability p_i = 0.9). Thus potency would be estimated at $\Sigma_o^i p_i k_i$, or 0.1(0) + 0.9(0.5) = 0.45. Future studies could yield J further estimates of potency, distributed perhaps between 0.4 and 0.6; the true potency is then given by summing the probability of these differing results—for example, 0.4(0.05) + 0.45(0.80) + 0.50(0.10) + 0.60(0.05) = 0.46. Finally, account must be taken of the likelihood of changing exercise behavior e_m; if we consider simply no increase of physical activity (e_o) and adoption of effective endurance training (e_i), the latter may have a probability of 0.5, so that the overall effectiveness E of the exercise tactic becomes 0.46(0.5) or 0.23.

Relevance to This Analysis

When Fentem and Bassey (1977) were asked by the British Department of Social Welfare to undertake an analysis of fitness economics, they concluded that it was premature to attempt any mathematical analysis. Instead, they contented themselves with presenting a concise "case for exercise."

The present report also recognizes the limitations of existing data. Nevertheless, as a stimulus to further research, it attempts to provide some answers to the various types of economic questions posed above, with a prime emphasis upon a cost-benefit justification of existing fitness programing. Given the favorable ratios for current programs, an obvious need exists to examine the merits of extending programing to a larger segment of the adult population.

Value Judgments

Avoiding value judgments is difficult. Philosophers, sociologists, and political scientists have long debated the virtues of a positivist philosophy, and some would consider cost-benefit analyses of recreational activity the ultimate nadir of enquiry (Fitch & Shanklin, 1970). Such calculations are nevertheless attractive at first inspection because difficult choices are then avoided—all decisions are reduced to a series of rational economic equations.

Certainly, possible policy alternatives can be weighed more logically and more intelligently if their respective costs are known. Nevertheless, excluding the question of cultural values from any economic discussion is difficult—indeed, values often determine the very framework of the questions we seek to solve. What is the purpose of a nation's economy? Is it to maximize the gross national product (GNP), or to assure the self-actualization of the individual citizen? Do we agree with Pope John Paul II (Encyclical On Human Work, 1981) concerning the "principle of the priority of labour over capital . . . labour is always a primary efficient cause, while capital, the whole collection of means of production, remains a mere instrument or instrumental cause"? We shall return to this issue of the person versus the capital that he or she can generate at several points in this monograph.

Factors Governing Health-Care Expenditures

Have health-care expenditures reached their logical ceiling? Some physicians would argue against any restriction of expensive operations such as coronary bypass surgery upon the grounds of age or adverse lifestyle, despite evidence that the money required for such surgical treatment could usefully be diverted to the prevention of coronary vascular disease in other members of the community. They would maintain that both the surgical and the preventive needs of the total population could be satisfied by increasing expenditures upon health and medical care.

Certainly the percentage of the gross national product devoted to health and medical care varies substantially from one nation to another (Fraser, 1983; Table 1.1). In Canada, expenditures have increased from 5.5% of the GNP in 1960 to 6.1% in 1965, 7.1% in 1970, 7.1% in 1975, and 8.3% in 1983 (Bennett & Krasny, 1981). Several lessons may be learned from such statistics. Gains of life expectancy are not directly proportional to medical expenditures. For example, in 1961 the British had a longer adult life expectancy than U.S. citizens, despite a much smaller expenditure on medical care (Table 1.2). Key variables are medical salaries, hospital operating costs, and uniformity of access to services. It also seems that many of the European social democracies are now approaching optimal expenditures, at least in terms of conventional medical services, and that a further outpouring of funds is having only a marginal effect upon life expectancy. At the same time it is arguable that some nations could afford a greater relative expenditure on health and medical care. Plainly,

Table 1.1 Health Care Expenditures Expressed as Percent of GNP—A Comparison of Eight "Western" Nations

Nation	1965 %	1965 Rank	1970 %	1970 Rank	1975 %	1975 Rank	1978 %
West Germany	5.2	5	6.1	6	9.7	1	
Sweden	5.8	4	7.5	1	8.7	2	
Netherlands	5.0	8	6.3	5	8.6	3	
USA	5.9	2	7.2	2	8.4	4	8.9
France	5.9	2	6.6	4	8.1	5	
Canada	6.1	1	7.1	3	7.1	6	7.0
Australia	5.2	5	5.6	8	7.0	7	
Finland	5.2	5	5.9	7	6.8	8	
United Kingdom	3.9	9	4.9	9	5.6	9	
Average	5.4		6.4		7.8		8.0

Note. From "Health Care Expenditures in Nine Industrialized Countries, 1960-1976" by J.G. Simanis and J.R. Coleman, 1980, *Social Security Bulletin*, **43**, pp. 3-8, and "Perspectives on Health" by J. Ableson, P. Paddon, and C. Strohmenger, 1983, Ottawa, Ministry of Supply and Services Occasional Paper, 82-504E.

Table 1.2 Life Expectancy at Age 15 Years—Data for Countries of Table 1.1 in 1961 and 1977

Country	Males 1961	Males 1977	% Gain	Females 1961	Females 1977	% Gain
West Germany	55.0	55.5	0.9	60.0	61.8	3.0
Sweden	58.5	58.8	0.5	61.9	65.0	5.0
Netherlands	58.3	58.4	0.2	62.4	64.8	3.8
USA	54.3	56.0	3.1	60.5	63.7	5.3
France	54.6	56.1	2.7	60.9	64.1	5.3
Canada	56.2	57.0	1.4	61.5	64.5	4.9
Australia	55.1	56.4	2.4	61.0	63.2	3.6
Finland	52.5	53.7	2.3	59.0	62.3	5.6
United Kingdom	55.3	56.7	2.5	60.8	62.6	3.0

Note. Based on data from the World Health Organization, from *World Health Statistics Annual*, 1980, Geneva: WHO, and on data from the United Nations, from *Demographic Yearbook, Special Issue: Historical Supplement*, 1979, New York: United Nations.

value judgments must be made. How much health and medical care can a given country afford relative to other social priorities, and how should funds be apportioned between active treatment (salaries of traditional clinicians, provision of hospital beds) and prevention?

One significant variable governing current medical expenditures is growth of the gross domestic product (GDP). In this respect, some nations have had a much more favorable recent experience than others. For example, between 1960 and 1977, the Japanese GDP increased by 233%, while that of Canada grew by only 77% (Fraser, 1983). Also, the public is realizing increasingly that a few individuals (and therefore a politically vulnerable group) are responsible for the current alarming costs of active medical treatment. In any 1 year, no more than 10% of the population enter hospitals; of this group, 87% are "low-cost" users, but 13% are recidivists, who account for 50% of all hospital costs (Zuk & Moore, 1980). It is hardly surprising that society has a growing ill-feeling toward the 1.3% of "big spenders" (i.e., 13% of 10%).

At the same time, health differs from many other socially purchased commodities. We have an interest in maintaining or restoring the health of our neighbors because we would like them to work for us, we are afraid of catching diseases from them, and we feel uncomfortable if we see them suffering (Drummond & Mooney, 1982). Indeed, some people regard life and health as priceless values that should not be measured in monetary terms (Waaler & Hjort, 1982).

Allocating Benefits to Reflect Different Values

Value judgments are made when benefits are allocated between various potential recipients (Muir-Gray, 1979). Let us suppose that fitness promotion allows a retiree to live to the age of 75 rather than 70 years. How much value should we impute to these added years? The individual and his or her immediate relatives would probably place a high value upon such an extension of life, but society as a whole might opt for the sparing of a younger and more "productive" individual.

Who Has the Authority to Choose?

The need for difficult budgetary decisions poses a major problem for society. Who should decide upon priorities? Does some elite know "what is best"? Is it reasonable to allow the "consumer" the right to choose lifestyle when he or she is not fully aware of either the advantages or the dangers of a particular type of behavior?

Decisions about health may be made by professionals (who have relevant expertise but also vested interests in specific solutions), parliamentarians (who may be strongly influenced by pressure groups in marginal constituencies), or the lay public (who tend to be ill-informed and vulnerable to the powerful forces of commercial advertising). While an absolute scale of values such as the Christian ethic, the Kantian moral imperative, or the "golden rule" might be sought, governmental policies in the long run will be decided by the electorate.

Relevance to This Analysis

Values will be discussed briefly where appropriate from the perspective of a physician with an interest in exercise as preventive therapy. However, the main focus of the present monograph will be upon the easier issues of cost/benefit and cost-effectiveness.

Cost Equivalence

In order to make valid calculations and comparisons, all costs must be translated to a common currency. The unit chosen for this purpose is the June 1983 Canadian dollar (Cdn. $1.00 = US $0.80 = £ Sterling 0.55). Economists have devised several techniques of measuring changes in the value of national currencies—the consumer price index, the producer price index, the chain price index for personal consumption expenditures, and the implicit price deflator for personal consumption expenditures. Substantial discrepancies exist between the various indices over the short term (1-2 years), but long-term changes (20-30 years) are more nearly comparable.

Calculations in this book are based upon the consumer price index (CPI). This indicates the current price of a "fixed" basket of goods and services as purchased by an urban consumer. Note that the content of the "basket" is inevitably a value judgment, and indeed the items to be purchased have been modified occasionally over the past 20 years.

Statistics for Canada and the U.S. are summarized in Table 1.3. Equivalent data for other countries has been taken from European Economic Community and U.N. handbooks. Several further considerations, now to be discussed, limit interpretations based on such a simple scaling of costs. Ideally, all important expenditures should be redetermined for the current year.

Shifts in Population Profile

The population of both Canada and the U.S. has grown substantially since 1960, and most items of national expenditure have experienced a roughly proportional change. The resultant difficulty in comparing suc-

Table 1.3 Changes in Purchasing Power of Canadian and U.S. Currency Between 1960 and 1983, as Estimated by Consumer Price Index

Year	Canadian Currency			U.S. Currency	
	Value of Canadian Dollar (1971 = 1.00)	Per Capita Health Expenditures (Fed./Prov./Municipal)		Value of U.S. Dollar (1971 = 1.00)	Medical Consumer Dollar
		Current Dollar	Constant Dollar		
1960	1.346			1.368	1.623
1961	1.333			1.354	1.577
1962	1.319			1.340	1.538
1963	1.295			1.324	1.500
1964	1.274			1.306	1.471
1965	1.242			1.284	1.435
1966	1.198			1.249	1.375
1967	1.156			1.214	1.284
1968	1.111			1.165	1.210
1969	1.062			1.106	1.132
1970	1.029			1.044	1.065
1971	1.000	198	198	1.000	1.000
1972	0.954	226	216	0.970	0.969
1973	0.887	257	228	0.913	0.932
1974	0.800	285	228	0.823	0.853
1975	0.722	346	250	0.754	0.762
1976	0.672	394	265	0.712	0.695
1977	0.622	441	274	0.669	0.634
1978	0.571	495	283	0.621	0.585
1979	0.523			0.559	0.536
1980	0.471			0.493	0.483
1981	0.419			0.451	0.444
1982	0.378			0.425	—
1983	0.357			0.409	—

Note. From *Canada Year Books*, Ottawa: Statistics Canada, and Statistical Abstracts of the United States, Washington, DC: U.S. Department of Commerce.

cessive years can be largely overcome by expressing data per adult or per employed worker.

The age distribution of the population is also altering (Shephard, 1978). A rising proportion of older adults has changed the pattern of health-care costs and increased the total demand for medical services. This trend will accelerate over the next two decades, and its effects will be enhanced because, in the future, most young women will be entering the labor force rather than caring for elderly parents in the way that earlier generations did.

Over the next few years, the proportion of dependent children will continue to decrease, and (probably) a marked change in family structures will become apparent (chapter 3). The first of these two changes may provide society with some opportunity to meet the growth of medical expenditures through a reduction of the education budget (Foot, 1982), but an increasing need to re-educate older adults will also occur. Future predictions are complicated by uncertainty regarding (a) the "opportunity cost" of children and thus the birth rate (Easterlin, 1978; Butz & Ward, 1978) and (b) the number, age, and skills of people moving from one country to another (Davies, 1977; Sawyer, 1979).

While old people are generally more vulnerable to illness than their younger counterparts, changes of lifestyle and advances in medical treatment have led to a significant waning of some diseases. For instance, the death rate for ischemic heart disease in North America among individuals of any given age has decreased over 30% since the mid-1960s (Walker, 1977; Anderson & Halliday, 1979). Aging and the waning of disease tend to cancel one another out (see Table 1.4). In the specific example of Table 1.4, the population mortality for cardiovascular disease decreased by only 13% despite a much larger decrease in the age-specific cardiovascular death rate.

Other secular trends relate to cigarette consumption, alcohol consumption, and annual vehicle mileage driven. All three of these risk

Table 1.4 Combined Impact of an Aging Population and a Declining Cardiovascular Mortality Upon the Incidence of Cardiac Fatalities—Illustrative Calculation for Male Subjects

Age (Years)	Data for 1962			Data for 1983			
	Mortality per 1000	Percent of Population	M × P	Mortality Change %	New Rate per 1000	Percent of Population	M × P
35-64	2.9	42.8	124.1	−26.0	2.15	41.8	89.9
65-74	14.6	4.94	72.1	−25.3	10.91	6.52	71.1
75-84	24.7	1.99	49.2	−12.8	21.54	2.62	56.4
<85	~35	0.27	9.5	−19.3	28.25	0.36	10.2
	Average mortality 5.10 per 1000			Average mortality 4.44 per 1000			

Note. From "Changing United States Life-Style and Declining Vascular Mortality: Cause or Coincidence?" by D.D. Walher, 1977, *New England Journal of Medicine, 297*, p. 164, and from "Changing Incidence of Disease" by G. Rose, 1970, in R.J. Jones (Ed.), *Atherosclerosis: Proceedings of the Second Inernational Symposium* (p. 312), New York: Springer, and from "The Aged and Society" by D. Wedderburn, 1973, in J.C. Brocklehurst (Ed.), *Textbook of Geriatric Medicine and Gerontology* (pp. 692-717), Edinburgh: Churchill-Livingstone.

factors have risen steeply in western nations over the past several decades and have had potentially adverse effects upon health; fortunately, evidence suggests that in many of the western nations, the epidemic of cigarette smoking has now passed its peak.

Measures of Productivity

Although differences of economic performance between the various industrialized nations have existed, the productivity and gross national product of most countries have shown sizable real gains over the past three decades; in Canada, the constant dollar GNP has grown almost fourfold in this time span. A given "constant dollar" expenditure thus has a differing social significance at different points in history. Most economists predict a slowing in the real growth of productivity over the next two decades. However, much depends upon the pace of technical change and the willingness of society to make real net investments to exploit available new technology. Aubry and Fleurent (1980) argued that an aging population may lead to an increase of personal savings during the next 20 years. On the debit side of the ledger, the aging labor force may also be limited by decreasing physical strength, impaired mobility, and obsolescence of human capital (formal education and training; Clark, Krebs, & Spengler, 1978; Espenschade & Serow, 1978; Thurow, 1980). Changes of productivity are less critical to the present analysis if we assume at least a temporary plateau of economic growth.

Differential Inflation

The statistics of Table 1.3 indicate the overall rate of inflation, but for accurate interpretation of earlier data, specific inflation rates covering individual costs and benefits must be calculated. For example, the general Canadian inflation rate for the period 1972-1982 was 150%, but the increase in the cost of recreational goods and services was much smaller (home recreation equipment, 69%; bicycles, 83%).* On the other hand, the inflation of medical and health-care costs substantially out-paced overall inflation (Harris, 1983, March 12); personal health care expenditures rose by a factor of 4.73 from 1960-1975 (unpublished data from Health and Welfare Canada).

---

*Note. The "real" increase in bicycle prices was probably larger than 83%, because between 1972 and 1982 many previously optional gadgets and luxury features were incorporated into the base price.

Differential Exchange Rates and Differential Pricing

In the U.S., the "shelter" component of the consumer price index is based on the cost of buying a house, while in Canada the corresponding item is the cost of residential accommodation. The U.S. statistic thus moves ahead of the Canadian CPI when interest rates are high and lags behind it when interest rates fall (Harris, 1983, March 12). Unfortunately, the real costs of many goods and services cannot be translated across national boundaries on such a simple basis as the CPI. Many items of sport equipment are cheaper in the U.S. than in Canada because of a larger market, while certain medical items and health-care products can be 2-3 times more costly a few miles south of the border.

The Trend Toward Urbanization

Over the past 3 decades, most national populations have shifted toward major urban centers. Residential densities are ever-increasing, and personal, private open space is rapidly disappearing. In the absence of corrective measures by appropriate levels of government, the future will likely hold an ever-increasingly passive pattern of indoor leisure and electronic entertainment. The trend toward total inactivity will be further exacerbated by displacement of work to the home through the use of video terminals.

Rapid escalation of land prices, associated with the changing urban structure of North American cities, has greatly increased the cost of providing facilities to sustain fitness, and in the absence of vigorous controls the rise of land values seems likely to continue.

These complex changes not only hamper the interpretation of old data, but they also make future extrapolations uncertain. Rising fuel costs will be one of several factors exacerbating the present migration of the population to medium and large cities, but this tendency may be offset by home employment, an increase of leisure time, or a lack of work opportunities in the large metropolises.

Relevance to This Analysis

The adoption of a common currency (1983 Canadian dollars) simplifies comparisons both between various countries and with other periods of world history. Nevertheless, such comparisons must take due account of changing population profiles, including such factors as age, ethnicity, and family structure. Any given dollar expenditure must be related to the Gross National Product of the country in question and due allowance must be made for differences of international exchange rates and commodity prices. Finally, all expenditures must be examined within the context of an increasingly urban society.

Accounting Conventions

A number of specific accounting conventions are applied in calculating the costs of illness (Klarman, 1981). These merit critical analysis.

Level of Employment

When estimating "lost" years of work due to death or morbidity, it is necessary to make assumptions about an individual's behavior if good health had prevailed. Unemployment is set at an arbitrary "normal" rate (4% in older U.S. papers, 5% in more recent investigations). Possibly, even the latter figure is unrealistically low for western nations over the next 2 decades. If so, "lost" earnings will be overestimated.

Adjustment is also needed for the anticipated participation of the population in the labor force (Table 1.5). Currently, about 97% of Canadian men participate over the age span 25-44 years, but the figure drops to 88% for those aged 45-64 years, and to 80% for all men over the age of 25. Female participation rates are much lower. Again, charting the future is difficult (Denton, Feaver, & Spencer, 1980; Foot, 1981). If opportunities for work further diminish, many companies may actively encourage employees to seek early retirement. This would reduce the potential economic gains from any type of health promotion program. Conversely, if an aging population, rampant inflation, or changes in retirement legislation extended the average number of working years, the economic gains from health promotion would increase.

The U.S. is currently enacting legislation to raise the retirement age from 65 to 67 years, effective in the year 2017, while the retirement age in some of the state socialist countries of Eastern Europe is as low as 57 years.

In most types of calculation, allowance must be made for the services of full-time homemakers. Usually, the value of a homemaker is assessed conservatively at the equivalent of a full-time domestic servant. If the real value were twice as large, with 20% of spouses continuing in a homemaking role, "lost" earnings would be underestimated by 10%.

Table 1.5 Average Income and Average Value per Person

Age (Years)	Average Income From Employment ($)	Participation in Labor Force (%)	Employment Rate (%)	Average Income /Person/Year ($)	Average Value /Person/Year ($)
Males					
20-24	12,389	86.1	90.5	9,654	2,415
25-34	22,434	97.0	95.9	20,868	5,217
35-44	27,395	97.0	95.9	25,484	6,371
45-54	27,438	88.3	96.1	23,283	5,822
55-64	24,613	88.3	96.1	20,886	5,221
65+	21,876	17.9	100.0	3,916	979
Females					
20-24	8,969	86.1	93.4	7,213	1,803
25-34	10,972	97.0	96.2	10,239	2,560
35-44	10,815	97.0	96.2	10,091	2,522
45-54	11,603	88.3	97.4	9,979	2,495
55-64	12,553	88.3	97.4	10,797	2,699
65+	15,055	17.9	100.0	2,695	674

Given three months absence from work per incident of coronary disease, the morbidity cost equals the average value per person. The mortality cost is the discounted average value, summed to retirement. Female participation in paid work is lower than for males. However, it is here assumed equal to male participation, as a means of including the worth of a full-time homemaker; in this calculation, homemakers have been allowed the same salary as other females of their age category.

Note. From The Relationships Between Physical Fitness and the Cost of Health Care (p. 22), Quasar, 1976, Toronto: Quasar Systems, Ltd.

Expressed in 1983 dollars.

Transfer Payments Between Sectors of the Economy

Fitness and recreational programing involves expenditures in at least four sectors of the economy (Martin & Mason, 1979)—the public sector (federal, state or provincial, regional and municipal governments, "nationalized" corporations), the commercial sector (sporting goods, facilities, services, employee fitness programs), the consumer sector (purchase of goods and services), and voluntary agencies. In many instances, these various forms of spending (and any resultant savings) overlap because they involve transfer payments from one sector to another. For example, commercial activity in producing sporting goods may stimulate consumer spending, will generate federal and state or provincial sales taxes, and may spur the support of voluntary organizations.

Economists generally exclude all transfer payments, including federal and provincial taxes, family allowances, and social security allowances from a cost-benefit balance sheet because these payments represent a "change in command" over the use of resources, rather than fresh earnings (Klarman, 1981). However, substantial sums of money are then neglected, and the resultant calculation of economic gain or loss gives no indication as to its distribution between the individual consumer, the corporate entrepreneur, and government.

One recent analysis for a commercial amusement park on the outskirts of Toronto (Table 1.6, Roberts & Wall, 1979) suggested that opening the new facility would transfer several million dollars from private pockets to government coffers through a combination of real estate and business taxes, provincial sales and amusement taxes, gasoline taxes, and income taxes. In contrast, if an individual becomes sick, government budgets are adversely affected by lost taxes, increased medical costs, and social security payments. Private enterprise will bear much of the associated burden of absenteeism, turnover, and lost productivity, while the individual family of a sick worker will lose wages and savings and carry a varying proportion of the direct medical expenses and many of the intangible costs discussed later.

Roberts (1982) estimated that in Australia, a combination of federal and state government and private medical insurance schemes shouldered 46% of the costs of cardiac disease, individual citizens carried 34.1%, and

Table 1.6 An Estimate of Revenues Transferred* to Various Levels of Government by Operation of a Theme Park ("Canada's Wonderland")

Level of Government	Without Park	With Park (T = Thousand)
Town of Vaughan	$ 3,636	$ 258 T
York Region	7,474	549 T
Province of Ontario	nil	3,232 T
Federal Government	nil	1,717 T
Total	$11,110	$5,756 T

*In this particular calculation, transfer payments are complicated by the possibility that part of the new revenue may come from foreign visitors. The transfer does not influence the world economy, but may benefit the national or the regional taxpayer.

Note. From "Possible Impacts of Vaughan Theme Park" by C. Roberts and G. Wall, 1979, *Recreational Research Review, 7*, p. 13.

Expressed in 1983 dollars for the year 1975.

others such as private employers met the remaining 19.9%. A rather similar distribution of costs may be anticipated in other developed nations.

Discounting Future Costs and Benefits

An attempt is usually made to discount future costs and benefits to their present day equivalents using such indices as the rate of return on long-term government bonds, the yield on industrial investments, or a social-time preference rate (a measure of national willingness to invest now for the benefit of future generations). Some early calculations used discount rates as low as 4%, but recent authors have adopted a higher figure; for example, Roberts (1982) assumed a "real" (constant dollar) interest rate of 8%. Weinstein (1983) has proposed converting the cost of a health initiative C into an equivalent annual stream C*, commencing in a future year f

$$C^* = rC (1 + r)^{f-o}$$

where r is the real (inflation corrected) discount rate. The lag period f depends on the time required to complete a study (L_1 years), to initiate action (L_2 years), and to obtain a biological response (W years):

$$f = L_1 + L_2 + W$$

For example, suppose we wish to justify an expensive longitudinal study of the benefits of physical activity. The study itself takes 10 years to complete (L_1 = 10 years). It then might take 5 years to change community habits (L_2 = 5 years), and in those people adopting increased exercise, a heart attack might be averted after an average of 10 years (L_3 = 10 years). The total lag period f is thus 25 years, and the cost to the community is not C (the figure requested by the investigator), but $C(1 + r)^f$. Assuming an interest rate of 8%, the cumulative cost at 25 years becomes 6.85C, and the corresponding *annual* cost is 0.08 (6.85C) or 55% of the sum requested!

Prediction of the discount rate over the next several decades is almost an impossibility—indeed, at the present juncture most economists hesitate to make 1-year predictions. It might thus be argued that major errors are inevitable when distant and putative benefits from a preventive program are evaluated. Although this is an important criticism of health-care economics during the phase of implementation, discounting can be neglected under "steady-state" conditions because each year a fresh cohort of the population avoids such contingencies as morbidity and premature death.

Cost of Premature Death

One major item in health-care balance sheets is the postponement of premature death. Some authors, such as Klarman (1981) and Rice (1966), calculate the resultant savings as gross earnings to the age of 65 years. Others, such as Weisbrod (1961), prefer estimating the added value attributable to an individual's employment, commonly taken to be 25% of gross earnings. A third approach equates the survival value of the individual with per capita gross domestic product (GDP) (Roberts, 1982). A final tactic, adopted in cost-effectiveness analysis, is to estimate total or quality-adjusted years of life purchased by a given dollar outlay.

Much depends upon personal philosophy. In general, economists can be divided into two camps—human capitalists and those interested in willingness to pay. The first school of thought considers humans as tools of production, placing no material value on the health of the very young and the elderly. This raises major ethical problems (Mooney, 1977; Waaler & Hjort, 1982) and, if carried to a logical conclusion, it would require superior health care for a high-salaried elite who was supposedly contributing the most to society—an unacceptable reincarnation of the master race philosophy.

An alternative viewpoint attempts to set some material value upon all members of society. Allowance of 100% of potential earnings during the period of employment plainly exaggerates the loss of human capital, but it has the merit of allowing some margin for the benefit of life beyond the age of 65 years. James Dowd (1975) was pessimistic when he wrote, "The aged have very little to exchange which is of any instrumental value. What skills they once had are outmoded; the skills which remain can often be provided more efficiently and with less cost by others." Nevertheless, survival is highly valued by the individual concerned, and by his or her immediate relatives. To cite Schelling (1968), "The life you save may be your own." While survival after retirement makes little direct contribution to a nation's wealth, important benefits may be transferred to the family and the immediate community—senior citizens serve as grandparents, foster grandparents, and academic tutors to the sick and the handicapped (Brooke, 1979; Murayama, 1979; Paillat, 1979; Streib & Streib, 1979).

Human capitalists also neglect social credits in the balance sheet, built up by the past contributions of the elderly to society. Some governments are now adopting a harsh economic line with retirees, denying them services available to younger individuals. For example, the British National Health Service has reportedly refused to provide renal dialysis to those over 65 years of age. However, fitness promotion is not concerned with the marginal extension of life by medical technology. It is aimed at adding years of healthy, fruitful living, and in this context no reason exists to discount longevity beyond the age of retirement.

The average gross domestic product gives a somewhat larger measure of the economic loss from premature death than do the earnings that are foregone (Krause, Gibbs, & Brown, 1977, December 28); the GDP reflects such factors as lost promotional opportunities, nursing care provided by the spouse, and inability to carry out minor domestic repairs and renovations. If the GDP approach is used, including the death or illness of full-time homemakers in the calculation is no longer appropriate (Roberts, 1982).

Intangible Costs

Some balance sheets incorporate an allowance for such intangibles as services purchased while sick, loss of income by spouse, grief, widowhood, and orphanhood. Unfortunately, no simple technique exists to measure the economic impact of such interpersonal problems. To date, investigators have either assumed that the intangibles represent a fixed percentage of other costs or have ignored these items.

Cost/Benefit Versus Cost-Effectiveness and Other Evaluation Methods

Program evaluation may follow an ordinal or a cardinal system (Whiting & Miller, 1977). With the ordinal approach (Smith, 1975), public input is used to establish a value system, which is then used to choose between various program alternatives. When a cardinal system is applied, costs and benefits, or effectiveness, are quantified, usually in dollar terms (Countryside Commission, 1977; Gibson, 1975; Neserow, Pompel, & Reich, 1975), and programs reaching an arbitrary cost-benefit ratio or cost-effectiveness ratio are approved.

Because of the many difficulties of completing analyses upon the costs and benefits of good health (including the major ethical dilemma of attributing zero value to the young and the elderly), a tendency among health economists has been to retreat to the less controversial ground of cost-effectiveness studies. Decisions can then be based on short-term behavioral changes without awaiting the results of lengthy (and ethically problematic) longitudinal studies. Items that can be examined are (a) the gross cost of a particular approach, (b) its total effect upon the economy (the multiplier effect), or (c) the willingness of the consumer to pay (the consumer surplus approach, based on the stated intentions of a population sample, or preferably demand behavior; Dwyer & Bowes, 1979). A total economic analysis also considers other items such as the influence of an exercise program upon property and commodity values (e.g., any change in housing prices near an urban fitness center, or in the yield of fish when a lake is opened for water sports).

In the context of health-effectiveness, we might inquire how large an investment in fitness promotion would be needed to assure a 50% success rate in controlling obesity or a 2-year extension of longevity in a middle-aged man with a high risk of coronary heart disease. Then there would be no need to impute any value to the control of obesity or the extension of life. Nevertheless, it would remain possible to compare the costs of fitness promotion with alternative approaches to treatment (such as psychotherapy for the obese, or smoking withdrawal for the coronary-prone).

If the decision has already been made to invest a fixed sum in preventive programs, a cost-effectiveness study might give useful guidance as to the best use of available dollars. However, only a cost-benefit analysis can give absolute justification to a program and show that it is adding to rather than subtracting from a national or a corporate exchequer. Cost-benefit analyses thus remain popular with both politicians and company presidents.

G. Kaplan (personal communication) has exploited the cost-effectiveness approach in his studies of chronic obstructive lung disease. His starting point has been that a 1-year extension of life obtained for $20,000 or less is worthwhile. If the cost is $20,000-$100,000, it becomes questionable, and if the cost exceeds $100,000, then the money is not well spent. Note that the sums involved are somewhat larger than average annual earnings and greatly exceed added capital.

If a person suffers considerable disability, the quality of life is rated at an appropriate proportion of unity (e.g., 0.5), and the effectiveness of treatment is adjusted accordingly (e.g., 2 years of survival at a quality of 0.5 is rated as a similar value to 1 year at a quality of 1.0).

An extension of this approach calculates health-status years. Each individual is ascribed an arbitrary life span of 100 years and achieves 100 health-status years if perfect health is maintained. Lesser allowances are accorded for life with one or more chronic conditions (multiplier of 0.74), with some limitation of activity (0.69), with limitation in the amount or kind of major activity (0.64), with inability to carry out major activities (0.57), or with permanent residence in a health-care institution (0.50). In mathematical terms, health-status years can be estimated as

$$_{t_o}\int^{T} \Sigma^{H}_{i=1} \ p_i i(t)v_i(t)\delta t$$

where p(t) is the probability of being in health state i at time t, v(t) is the multiplier for health state i at time t, H is the number of health states chosen for the calculation, t is the starting age, and T is the ending age.

Although they were developed by exponents of cost-effectiveness analysis, the methods proposed for partial disability can also be incorporated into cost-benefit analyses and are particularly helpful in the geriatric sector (chapter 6).

Evaluating Fitness Programing by Degree of Maturity

One analysis of methods used to date in justifying fitness and recreational expenditures (Nienaber & Wildavsky, 1973) suggested that the most popular tactic was a comparison with previously established standard expenditures. Unfortunately, such an approach neglects the natural history of governmental initiatives. Any fiscal review should take account of program maturation (Godin & Shephard, 1983) and appropriately progress from process through impact to outcome evaluation. Process and impact measures are susceptible to cost-effectiveness analysis.

In the context of fitness programing, possible process measures might include the number of facilities available and their physical attractiveness and data on the range and number of programs offered. Impact could be gauged from total attendance, participant hours, and the percentage of various social and ethnic groups that became involved in the programs. Outcome might examine the perceived life satisfaction of the population, the incidence of fitness-related illnesses, the safety of various program alternatives, indices of economic benefit (gains of business income, job opportunities, and property values), and various delinquency and crime rates (Hatry & Dunn, 1971).

While a program remains in the "embryonic" stage, considerable reliance must be placed on various types of process review from peer evaluations to audits of the activity undertaken. In the early days of any program, few users exist, and the participation growth rate is slow; major adaptations of structure are still necessary to allow efficient program delivery, and funding (for research, development, and program design) must be generous relative to effectiveness (as gauged from the emergence of a strong program).

A "growth" phase follows when program d
Participation increases rapidly. At this stage quite
be needed in many segments of the program to m;
ness. For example, an employee fitness program i
trants, but adjustment of working hours must be n
participation.

At "maturity," participation is approaching a
program developments that may be proposed are counterbalanced by the
curtailment or termination of less successful initiatives. In general, program changes are quite minor at this stage. The budgetary concern turns
from process to impact evaluation with a view to selecting emphases that
will assure a maximum penetration of the market. North American fitness programs are, in general, approaching this mature state. Existing
initiatives apparently serve some sectors of the community well, although
skeptics have pointed to poor compliance rates, questioning how long
health and industrial benefits are sustained. An urgent need exists for
programs that will reach target groups other than young adults of middle-
to high-socioeconomic status.

When "saturation" has been achieved, it becomes appropriate to
examine critically the financial resources that have been committed in
terms of benefits and fiscal efficiency and the governmental or managerial
division concerned that is arguing its needs relative to competing programs. Because portions of the fitness market (e.g., the elderly and the
disabled) have yet to be penetrated, outcome analysis arguably is premature. Moreover, the choice of outcome criteria remains debatable; some
commonly proposed indicators such as mortality rates require an excessively long period of prospective observation. More attractive alternatives
with a faster payoff include indices of morbidity and current health status
such as a health hazard index. Despite the current limitations of these
various statistics, justification remains for carrying out some preliminary
analyses using quite complex cost-benefit models. Such analyses provide
a basis for the more definitive work that will become possible with saturation of the fitness market.

Finally, some programs reach a phase of "privatization." If an operation is demonstrated as cost-beneficial not only to the nation but also
to the program operator, then transfer of a government-sponsored
initiative to the private sector of the economy can be considered. Key
queries at this late stage of a program are whether or not an orderly transfer of responsibility can be arranged, what an appropriate compensation
to government for its equity is, and whether or not private corporations
have the ability and desire to deliver the program efficiently to all sectors
of the target population.

ctics and Strategy

The following chapters will attempt to address the tactics and the strategy of fitness planning within the context of what seems to be a shrinking budgetary envelope. However, a recovery of international trade could quite rapidly reduce current fiscal constraints, and a disagreement remains concerning the medium- and long-term economic prospects for western society. In the short-term, program review should examine not only the cost side of the ledger, but also the potential of fitness programing to stimulate economic growth. It should also present information in such a fashion that it can be related to both economic priorities and urgent social concerns.

The ultimate source of revenue for any government or corporation is its labor force. Information on costs and benefits have thus been simplified by expressing all data in dollars per worker-year. Such units allow comparisons between companies and between nations, despite historic changes in the absolute and relative numbers of employed workers.

At many points costs will be presented with apparent precision, but it must be emphasized that in reality all estimates encompass a large margin of error. The limits of confidence are lacking for most variables, and for some components of the balance sheet even the method of calculation is disputed. Moreover, the cost-benefit ratio will inevitably change as penetration of the fitness market increases. Numbers are cited (a) to test the suggested methods of calculation, (b) to provide an approximate benchmark for the mid-1980s, and (c) to indicate areas of both cost and benefit that merit more detailed future research. Such statistics should be refined to the point where they are entirely credible to those making hard fiscal policy decisions and can be applied to individual components of budget planning, program delivery, and evaluation.

Conclusions

The conventional methodology of cost-benefit and cost-effectiveness analysis must take due account of reasons for costing (e.g., to assess the efficiency of existing programs or the effects of expanding services). Value judgments are unavoidable in making such decisions. Costs are standardized here in terms of 1983 Canadian dollars per worker-year, and such figures must be interpreted relative to secular trends in population profile, investment, and productivity.

chapter 2

Personal Consequences
of Enhanced Physical Fitness

"Ah quanta spes est, Lapidum sperare Sapientium!" What a hope that is, to have the Philosopher's Stone! Yet what shall it profit him if meanwhile he that has it sickens? . . . Yet none of these need the Chymist fear . . . this noble Medicine (has) the virtue of combatting all the embattled forces of disease—it sustains the very vitals, nourishes the breath, and so conserves the natural heat that perfusing the whole body and entering all the limbs it engenders and maintains there a constant motion and vigour. (Von Boerhaave, 1737)

From the personal point of view, regular physical activity involves a substantial expenditure of time by both participants and volunteer leaders. However, physical activity also brings physical and psychological benefits with a reduction in medical and rehabilitative costs. A physically fit person has a greater capacity to enjoy a full and robust lifestyle than does someone who is physically less fit. A more healthy pattern of nutrition may also be adopted with other beneficial changes of personal habits (including a correction of alcohol and tobacco abuse, stress control, and improved patterns of sleep). Finally, some evidence suggests that a growing child's learning process is helped.

Time Constraints

Any expenditure of leisure time involves an opportunity cost. This may be measured in terms of the foregone opportunities to pursue activity A if time is allocated to activity B. Alternatively, one can assess the income that is foregone. Thus the time that is spent in exercising or in traveling to and from an exercise facility can no longer be spent in other ways. Indeed, a dollar figure for this opportunity cost is often combined with more direct expenditures (admission fees and transportation costs) when assessing the demand for various forms of recreation (Vickerman, 1975; Smith, 1983).

Because most individuals are constrained to a fixed 30- or 40-hr working week, costing of opportunity in terms such as the average hourly wage is biased. Arguably, if Jones did not go jogging, he would have spent his evening slumped in front of a television set with a six-pack of beer. This statement in itself illustrates the potential economic impact of increased physical activity upon both the breweries and governmental revenues. A more general consequence of the opportunity expense associated with an increase in physical activity is that the demand for all forms of passive leisure entertainment (from spectator sports to movies, television, books, and magazines) will be reduced. This response is enhanced by a reallocation of disposable income as individuals become more active (see chapter 3).

Minimum Requirements of Time and Energy

Teenagers and young adults who train for international competitions invest many hours in daily practice and sustain tremendous opportunity costs in terms of foregone social and psychological development. The average citizen neither needs nor wants a commitment of this order; he or she is interested rather in the minimum requirement of time and energy to assure good health and generate the other economic benefits to be discussed later. Unfortunately, little agreement exists on an appropriate investment of time and energy, and how far an increase in the frequency and duration of exercise can compensate for any shortcomings in its intensity is not clear (Pollock, 1973; Shephard, 1975).

One fairly widely accepted recommendation is that a middle-aged adult should allocate five 30-min periods per week of vigorous large muscle activity to develop fitness and three 30-min periods per week to maintain fitness (Shephard, 1977b). For the purpose of the present analysis, this health need can be satisfied through vigorous endurance-type activities (e.g., jogging, cycling, swimming, or longer bouts of fast walking), well-organized employee fitness programs, and certain types of individual and team sports. Accordingly, the focus will be upon this type of physical activity. Nevertheless, an enormous variation remains in direct costs, opportunity costs, and economic benefits, depending upon the sort of endurance exercise that is chosen. Likewise, a tremendous interindividual variation exists in real and perceived disposable leisure.

One recent analysis of techniques for shedding 10 kg of fat recommends jogging rather than cycling, walking, or calisthenics on the basis that the joggers encounter a lower opportunity cost per kg of fat loss

(Rhodes, 1982, May). However, the opportunity cost would become even smaller if the necessary activity were incorporated into the routine of daily living. For example, a 30-min cycle ride to work might replace a car journey of at least a 20-min duration. If a quiet cycle path were available, it might even be possible to allocate some of the 30 min to planning the day's work so that the opportunity cost would drop to near zero. Alternatively, the exercise session might allow the enjoyment of a symphony through the use of a portable tape recorder and earphones. The next lowest opportunity cost is generally seen with an on-site employee fitness program. In such an arrangement, no appreciable time is lost in travel to and from the gymnasium. This represents a significant saving relative to many forms of active recreation in which the "travel space" is such that journey times may exceed exercise times by a factor of 2-5 (Cicchetti, 1973; Duffield, 1975; Marans & Fly, 1981; Smith, 1983).

Exercise enthusiasts generally place "convenience of facilities" fairly high on their list of priorities, although presumably the comparison is drawn between a nearby resource and a similar facility that is located at some distance. North Americans often bypass the nearest recreational location. Kates, Peat, Marwick and Co. (1970) developed a sophisticated mathematical model of recreational preferences that included assessments of the quality, the user costs, and the variety or complementarity of the facility in relation to personal income. Scope remains to apply this type of analysis to examine how far program organizers should accept an increase of opportunity costs in order to add variety to a conditioning regimen.

Disposable Leisure Time

Perceived leisure varies with personality type: for example, the Type A individual (Friedman & Rosenman, 1974) fills available minutes with a wide variety of pursuits. Arguably (although not yet demonstrated) the opportunity cost of active recreation is higher for a Type A than for a Type B individual. Then again, once convinced of the desirability of exercise, the Type A individual may be more willing than the Type B individual to spend the necessary time on maintaining fitness (Oldridge, 1979).

True leisure time varies widely from a few minutes to several hours per night and is affected by (a) the duration of paid work (including overtime and moonlighting), (b) the division of labor in the home, (c) daily travel time, and (d) the number and age of dependents. Average values are surprisingly similar for western democracies and communist states; statistics from East Germany show that women (3.3 hrs) have less free time than men (4.5 hrs), and participation in active sports lag far behind other recreational interests such as watching television, reading, dancing, and meeting with friends (Stundl, 1977; Hanke, 1979).

Costing Time

Some economists charge the opportunity cost of time foregone on a fixed scale such as the average wage ($10 • h^{-1}). But in reality, placing a consistent dollar value upon the opportunity cost of time invested in physical activity is difficult. This is a value judgment made by the individual, who weighs the merits of a given form of exercise against alternative uses of leisure. Nevertheless, establishing average opportunity costs that have significant negative impacts upon the utilization of a facility or a resource is possible. For example, recreational land in Ontario becomes unpopular when the price of a weekend by a lake exceeds 3 hrs of travel in each direction. The availability of such land could become an important issue if an increased proportion of the population were to seek outdoor recreation (chapter 3).

The opportunity costs associated with leisure time do not remain fixed from one generation to another. For example, during the Edwardian era, Sundays were devoted to attending church, and the weekly leisure time of most workers was limited to Saturday afternoons. Under such conditions, Torontonians found that within-city attractions such as the Sunnyside Amusement Park were more appropriate places to seek their weekend recreations than the lakeland of Muskoka, 200 km to the north. In the future it seems likely that automation and "structural unemployment" will leave much of the population with long periods of free time, effectively decreasing the opportunity costs for travel to and participation in physical activity (Levasseur & Bellefleur, 1976; Tremblay, 1976; Sue, 1982). In essence, time must be priced according to its scarcity value (Wilman, 1980). This has a bearing upon the possibility of exploiting wilderness recreation in remote locations (chapter 3). Improvements in road, rail, or air networks also reduce opportunity costs by shortening travel time (Anderson, 1975).

The Contribution of the Volunteer

Dauriac (1982) stressed the important contribution of the volunteer to sport programing in a comparison of data from Canada, France, and the U.S. In France, the number of individuals certified by 10 sport federations increased from 873,000 in 1955 to 2.2 million in 1970, and particularly large gains were reported by organizations for skiing (80,000 rising to 580,000) and judo (20,000 to 190,000) (Coronio & Muret, 1973). In Canada, 15.2% of the population over the age of 14 years provided various forms of volunteer service during 1980; 374 million hrs of such work included 51.6 million hrs related to sport (about 5.9 hrs per worker-year^{-1}, with a greater relative contribution from higher socioeconomic groups). Assessed at an average wage ($10 • h^{-1}), the value of volunteer sport and fitness leaders would be about $59 per worker-year^{-1}, ignoring travel time and other incidental contributions. However, governmental contributions to the housing and operation of voluntary sport governing bodies should be set against this apparently substantial resource. Thus the Province of Ontario contributes $7.3M per year (i.e., $61 per sport volunteer) to such agencies.

Not all of the $61 governmental contribution is spent in motivating and training volunteers, and such individuals plainly make a substantial net contribution to municipal and other levels of government. Nevertheless, it remains arguable that in the absence of fitness and sport programs, the same people would make an alternative contribution to other useful social needs. Berger (1983) noted that in Ontario, the current ranking of volunteer hours was social welfare (33%), religion (29%), leisure (20%), education (17%), health (8%), and other (15%); sport accounted for about 12.5% of the 20.0% leisure item. In other Canadian provinces, sport occupies an even larger percentage of the total volunteer time (e.g., 27% in Saskatchewan and 20% in Manitoba).

To date, most of the volunteer effort has been with organized sport, although potential exists for a similar contribution to programs with greater immediate impacts on fitness. Thus in the Canada Life employee fitness project (chapter 4), 6 volunteers provided about 18 hrs of fitness class leadership per week with an equivalent value of about $7200 per year, or $6 per company employee per year.

The individual's net investment in volunteer work may have a value of less than $10 • h^{-1} because the opportunity cost is usually matched through the important dividend of self-actualization. Occasionally the rewards sought by volunteers may be inappropriate, a situation less easily corrected with unpaid than with paid employees.

Berger (1983) estimated that in Ontario, 47¢ of volunteer effort was generated for every dollar invested in recreation programs by the provincial government.

Physical and Psychological Benefits

The physically active individual has a greater cardiorespiratory and muscular endurance than a sedentary person. Physical tasks around an urban home or a rural cottage are performed more readily and with a reduced sense of fatigue (Shephard, 1977b). The body has a more attractive appearance, and heat tolerance is improved. Stronger muscles also leave the individual at lesser risk of lower-back injuries and hernias, while greater flexibility enhances the possible range of pursuits for an older individual. Lastly, the absence of physical disability is a clear benefit that most individuals would value highly.

In essence, these are "opportunity dividends." Their dollar worths are a personal judgment, although techniques are now evolving whereby a subject can rate the perceived value of avoiding various types of medical disorders (Wolfson, 1974; Torrance, 1976) and can assign an approximate dollar figure to the conservation of specific health attributes (Plutchik, Conte, & Weiner, 1973). One criterion that could be applied to some physical benefits, such as a slim figure, is the price charged by commercial operations that promise the desired attribute. Presumably, the fee bears a relationship to perceived worth, at least for that segment of the market with a substantial disposable income.

Many people value physical activity because it makes them "feel better." Attempts to document this phenomenon have not been particularly successful (Shephard, 1983c). Possible causes of an elevated mood include a secretion of catecholamines or of endorphins by the brain (Farrell, Gates, Maskeid, & Morgan, 1982), an optimization of arousal, and some relief of mental stress (Layman, 1974). Again, these must be regarded as opportunity dividends, and they are difficult to quantify.

It has been suggested that such a phenomenon as exercise addiction exists (Sachs, 1982) with the development of a progressive dependence upon the production of endogenous morphine-like substances. If this is the case, a crude fiscal evaluation of the process might be derived from the analogy of dependence upon exogenous opiates. An addict of this sort pays $50-150 per day to sustain the habit. The analogy is extreme, but nevertheless, the person who chooses to spend several hours per day on distance running could conceivably earn $10-50 per hour if the same time were allocated to a commercial endeavor, while the direct costs of distance running can sometimes rise to $5000-6000 per year (chapter 6).

Medical and Rehabilitative Costs

Escalating medical and health-care costs are a major concern throughout the western world (Squires, 1982; Brennan, 1982a). The response of the federal and state or provincial governments has generally been a compression of budgets for education, universities, and transportation over the past decade (Cappon, 1983, March/April). U.S. experts have also encouraged innovative methods of health-care funding and regulation of benefits (Rogers, Eaton, & Bruhn, 1981). Part of the U.S. burden of medical costs is passed to both domestic and foreign consumers of manufactured goods. Thus Roccella (1982) estimated that provision for medical and health-care payments added the current equivalent of $237 to the Canadian purchase price of an average Ford car, while at General Motors the medical premium was $294 per vehicle. Other exports from the U.S. presumably carry a medical tax of similar order depending upon the labor content of the item purchased.

The overall cost of illness in the U.S. has been estimated at the annual equivalent of Canadian $623 billion, or about $5460 per wage earner per year. The balance sheet includes direct costs of $280.7B (hospitalization, physician visits, medications) plus indirect costs of $136.2B for morbidity and $206.6B for premature death. In keeping with the philosophy of Klarman (1981), the U.S. statistics allow lost earnings at 100% of value, but make no allowance for intangible costs. The proportion of U.S. federal health expenditures allocated to preventive tactics has been estimated at 2.6% (Thomas, 1979) to 4% (U.S. Surgeon General, 1979) of the available budget.

Roberts (1982) set Australian direct costs of illness at the equivalent of $12.1B per year, $1375 per wage earner per year. He noted that the items relevant to cardiovascular disease included hospital services ($5.13B), ambulance services ($0.16B), pharmaceuticals ($1.15B), and medical services ($2.09B).

The calculations of Quasar (1976) for the Province of Ontario present some interesting contrasts with both the U.S. and the Australian calculations (Table 2.1). The Quasar estimate includes dental services but excludes expenditures for medical education and research. Likewise, it excludes intangibles from the indirect costs. The grand total of $8.37B amounts to $1915 per adult per year, or $3054 per wage earner per year. The discrepancy from the U.S. analysis is largely attributable to a smaller allowance for the costs of premature mortality (25% rather than 100% of earnings). If 100% of earnings had been imputed, the annual cost would have increased to $5573 per wage earner. The close agreement of the latter figure with the U.S. estimate remains fortuitous because the Ontario morbidity statistics reflect days of hospital admission rather than total days of illness.

In 1978 (Wilkins & Adams, 1983), 0.9% of Canadians were residents of long-term health-care institutions (homes for the aged, retarded or physically handicapped, and chronic care and mental hospitals), a further 2.1% suffered sufficient disability that they were chronically unable to work, attend school, or keep house, and 7.1% were "somewhat restricted." An additional 2.2% had health problems that usually restricted

Table 2.1 Direct and Indirect Costs of Coronary Heart Disease in the Province of Ontario

Cost	(M = Million)
Direct costs	
Hospital services	$ 497M
Physicians' services	116M
Pharmaceuticals	116M
Medical education and research	Excluded
Total	$ 729M
Indirect costs	
Total	$ 744M
Grand total (direct and indirect costs)	$1473M
($538 per worker-year)	

Note. From *The Relationships Between Physical Fitness and the Cost of Health Care* (p. 11) by Quasar, 1976, Toronto: Quasar Systems, Ltd.
Expressed in 1983 Canadian dollars.

recreation or community functions, and 2.0% were temporarily disabled by illness or accidents.

While argument will continue regarding the detailed costing of illness and disability, it must be accepted that the annual burden is very large (20-30% of an average income). Moreover, about half of the total costs of illness and disability (10-15% of an average income) are susceptible to preventive tactics, and at least a quarter of the total reflect lifestyle items (Table 2.2) such as physical inactivity and the abuse of alcohol and tobacco (Fletcher, 1959; Berry & Boland, 1977; Luce & Schweitzer, 1978).

Several analyses from the U.S. have stressed the impact of absenteeism upon corporate profitability. Absences ascribed to illness cost the U.S. economy at least 132 million days of work per year, while 70% of the U.S. labor force have debilitating back pains at some point in their careers (T. Albright—personal communication). American business pays approximately 25% of U.S. costs for medical and health care. At Citibank, current charges are $1936 per employee, while at New York Telephone the bill for medical costs is about $300M per year, or $3731 per worker.

Participation Rates

The impact of any fitness or exercise program depends heavily on (a) how many people are attracted to it, (b) whether those who are re-

Table 2.2 Estimated Direct Costs of Illnesses Related to Modern Lifestyle

Disorder	Direct Cost (M = Million)	Effect of Exercise Direct	Indirect
Neoplasms (Cancers of upper digestive system, lungs, and other respiratory organs)	$ 31.6M	—	?
Metabolic diseases (Obesity, gout)	16.1M	+	—
Mental disorders (Alcoholic psychosis, alcoholism, drug dependence, personality disorders)	102.9M	—	?
Circulatory disorders (Except rheumatic fever and rheumatic heart disease)	569.1M	+	—
Diseases of digestive system (Hernias, cirrhosis)	89.4M	—	?
Musculoskeletal diseases (Osteoarthritis, bursitis, rheumatism, synovitis, inter-vertebral disc displacement, knee derangement, joint dislocation)	148.4M	—	?
Accidents, poisoning, violence	347.4M	—	?
Total	$1304.9M		
Percentage of Ontario total	29.2%		
Directly affected by exercise	13.1%		
Possible indirect effect of exercise	16.1%		

Note. From *The Relationships Between Physical Fitness and the Cost of Health Care* (p. 9) by Quasar, 1976, Toronto: Quasar Systems, Ltd.

Expressed in 1983 dollars.

cruited were active previously, and (c) whether they are drawn from the healthy or the unhealthy segment of the community.

Calculations throughout this report are based on the assumption that 20% of the labor force will participate in well-designed physical activity classes. Current U.S. and Canadian experience suggests that 40-50% of employees will begin an "on-site" program (Shephard, 1979; Shephard, Cox, & Corey, 1981; Marsden & Youlden, 1979; Beck, 1982; Fielding, 1982); but it also suggests that "steady-state" adherence is generally no better than 20% (Yarvote, McDonagh, & Goldman, 1974; Cox, Shephard, & Corey, 1981; Song, Shephard, & Cox, 1982; Andresky, 1982, December). At the Exxon Corporation 65% of executives initially recruited to a fitness facility were still exercising two or more times per week after 1 year (Yarvote et al., 1974), but at NASA only 38.4% continued to exercise 2 or more days per week (Durbeck et al., 1972). Critics have further stressed that the published adherence rates refer largely to white-collar groups, often drawn from health-related types of employment (insurance companies and hospitals). Even in such populations, the regular use of off-site facilities is lower than the use of company-sponsored programs at the workplace. No more than 10-25% of employees are even recruited with such an arrangement (Fielding, 1982).

In both the Toronto Life Assurance program and the General Foods program (chapter 4), at least a quarter of participants were previously active elsewhere. However, previously active individuals have not been discounted here, because continuing health benefits are assured by attendance at the employee fitness program.

The type of individual who is recruited into an activity program is often health-conscious; subsequent attrition of participants can lead to an accentuation of this bias because obese workers and smokers defect from the program (Massie & Shephard, 1971; Sidney & Shephard, 1976). However, experience with the Toronto Life Assurance program suggests that, with suitable recruitment propaganda and an appropriately graded progression of training, this bias need not develop. Accordingly, no discount has been applied for a selective recruitment of fit participants. Critical observers will appreciate that selectivity of recruitment, and sample attrition is an important fiscal limitation of many programs that merits further investigation. Other aspects of the participation rate are considered in chapter 3.

Acute Illness

The burden of acute illness could be modified by an effect of exercise upon immune responses, lifestyle, or mood.

Occasional reports claim that exhausting exercise increases a person's susceptibility to acute bacterial and viral infections through a stress reaction (Selye, 1974). Early authors found that physical activity had little effect upon immune function (see Jokl, 1931, 1977 for reviews), but some more recent articles have suggested that prolonged exercise increases the number of T lymphocytes (Steel, Evans, & Smith, 1974), B lymphocytes (Hedfords, Holm, & Ohnell, 1976), and polymorphs (Eskola et al., 1978). Thirty minutes after exercise, cortisol levels are increased, the white cell population drops, and a decreased ability to clear the blood of bacterial particles is apparent (Matracia & Matracia, 1980). Apparently, if exercise is stressful enough to increase the output of hydrocortisone, it interferes with the availability of Fc receptors on the neutrophils, which restricts ingestion of immunoglobulin G sensitized particles (Klempner & Gallin, 1978). Exercise may also induce acute changes in the type of phagocytic cells circulating in the blood (Bellina, Savalla, Caruso, & Matracia, 1980; Cillari, Gargano, Bellavia, & Matracia, 1980). Such responses could conceivably modify acute reactions to microorganisms. On the other hand, the overall immune function appears to be unchanged by several months of regular vigorous training (Mazza, 1980).

While it can be concluded that immune function is essentially unaltered as an individual improves in fitness, the average duration of an acute infection is nevertheless substantially influenced by lifestyle patterns. To take a specific example, the habit of heavy cigarette smoking doubles the duration of symptoms and physiological disturbances following an acute upper-respiratory infection. Bed rest and disability days are also about twice as long for a smoker as for a nonsmoker (Editor, British Medical Journal, 1974). To the extent that exercise facilitates both the process of smoking withdrawal and other improvements of lifestyle, it corrects the charges imposed upon the national economy by adverse health habits.

The possibility that participation in a program of vigorous physical activity will improve perceived health is of great practical importance (Kohn & White, 1976). Behavioral scientists recognize increasingly that no sharp boundary exists between health and disease (Herzlich, 1973; Sackett, Chambers, MacPherson, Goldsmith, & McAuley, 1977; Chambers, 1982). Many if not most absences from duty and many if not most medical consultations lack any clear organic causes. Berger (1983) suggested that psychiatric problems were responsible for at least 60% of absenteeism, while 80-90% of industrial accidents and 65-80% of dismissals were for personal problems. Thus much of the current burden of minor ill-health and poor industrial performance might disappear if workers felt better and attained the state of "complete mental, physical, and social well-being" that the World Health Organization (1948) defines as *health*. Notably, one of the most common reasons cited for exercising is "to feel better." Some (Morgan & Horstman, 1976; Michael, 1957; Lion, 1978; Folkins, 1976; Pauly, Palmer, Wright, & Pfeiffer, 1982), but not all (Massie & Shephard, 1971; Young & Ismail, 1976) authors have found reductions of anxiety with regular exercise. Other investigators (Hughes, 1974; Henderson, 1974; White, 1974; Pauly et al., 1982; but not Leonardson & Garguilo, 1978; nor Gary & Guthrie, 1972) have also commented on improvements in self-concept through regular physical activity. The potential fiscal benefits of psychological health are large. One recent analysis put the costs of stress alone at $4107 per affected worker; the author of the report in question further suggested that such charges could be reduced to $600-700 per affected individual if the stress received optimal treatment (Manuso, 1983).

Both cross-sectional studies (Palmore, 1970; Cheraskin & Ringsdorf, 1973) and a longitudinal experiment (Sidney & Shephard, 1976) support the concept that exercise contributes to well-being; relationships exist between regular physical activity, an improvement of perceived health, and a decreased incidence of vague miscellaneous diseases in middle-aged and older adults. Wiley and Camacho (1980) applied an overall measure of health status to the residents of Alameda County, CA. Even excluding those with chronic disabilities, a strong association existed between moderate physical activity and health status.

A controlled longitudinal experiment with Quebecois primary school students (Shephard, 1982a) showed that 5 hrs of additional physical activity per week actually *increased* the absenteeism of 6-year-olds by 3 days per year (from 10 to 13 days per year). However, in students aged 7-12 years, absenteeism was the same for exercised and control samples (each group missed 4 days of school per year, substantially less than the usual rate of industrial absenteeism). These findings suggest that parents were unwilling to expose very young children to a combination of the school exercise program and some minor infection. Nevertheless, neither immune function nor the child's perception of his or her own health was changed by the daily hour of vigorous activity, so school attendance became comparable in exercised and control groups once the age of over-protection was past. The absenteeism of 6-year-old children undoubtedly had some impact on the work habits of their mothers. Currently, only about 50% of mothers are employed outside the home, but some economists predict that labor-force participation rates for this group will rise to 80% in the near future. Suppose that all children followed the required activity program and 80% of the mothers worked while caring for an average of 2 children. The total work-loss attributable to an adverse effect on the school attendance of 6-year-olds would then amount to an average of 6 days per family, affecting 80/180% of the labor force. Also, assuming a working span of 40 years and a 1.75-fold replacement cost for missing labor,* the average cost would be 0.117 days per year. Given 220 days of work per year, at a salary of $14,500, the annual cost of this item would become $7.70 per employed worker.

The personal value of fewer acute infections and an optimization of health is highly subjective. At present, no simple method of introducing

---

Note. A replacement cost of greater than unity is necessary for several reasons: (a) Absences are unpredictable, so a margin of labor must be held in reserve; (b) shortfalls of production may lead to overtime work; and (c) the replacement is generally less well-trained and therefore less efficient at the required task (see further chapter 1).

such an item into our balance sheet exists. Economic consequences of changes in morbidity and perceived health are reflected in the calculations of health insurance payments and absenteeism.

Chronic Illness

Accumulated evidence shows that regular physical activity has preventive value in a wide range of chronic medical conditions, including ischemic heart disease (Morris et al., 1973; Paffenbarger, 1977; Paffenbarger, Wing, & Hyde, 1978; Shephard, 1981), hypertension (with its associated renal and cerebrovascular complications (Kukkonen, Rauramaa, Voutilainen, & Länsimies, 1982a), peripheral vascular disease such as arteriosclerosis (Isacsson, 1972), obesity (with the associated problems of diabetes, cholecystitis, hypertension, and renal disorders) (Shephard, 1977b), asthma (Shephard, 1982a; Kukkonen, Rauramaa, Siitonen, & Hänninen, 1982b), back and knee injuries, bone demineralization (Smith & Babcock, 1973), and certain mental disorders. Furthermore, a progressive, exercise-centered rehabilitation program shortens the period of disability once symptoms have appeared in patients who are limited by bed rest, ischemic heart disease (myocardial infarction and/or angina), hypertension and stroke, peripheral vascular disease with claudicant pain, diabetes, asthma, cystic fibrosis, chronic obstructive lung disease, physical injury, rheumatoid arthritis, and osteoarthritis (Shephard, 1978).

Modification of chronic illness has economic value mainly because it improves the quality of life; ideally, everyone would live a disability-free life until the day of death. Circulatory diseases are the main category of illnesses directly affected by exercise (Table 2.2). Statistics from the Province of Ontario (Quasar, 1976) show that circulatory disorders account for 12.9% of direct costs and 21.7% of indirect costs, or, on the 25% "added value" hypothesis, 17.6% of all costs of illness.

Good evidence exists to show that an increase of physical activity approximately halves the risk of subsequent coronary disease (Tables 2.3-2.6). The costs of premature death will be considered later, but direct personal and impersonal costs of heart disease remain (such as hospital and physician services), as do losses of output from morbidity and intangibles such as grief. Klarman (1964) estimated that these items cost the U.S. ($3.1B + 8.2B) in 1962. Their current worth would be about $47.1B, or, given a U.S. labor force of 110 million, $428 per worker-year. If vigorous exercise halved this cost and 20% of workers and their spouses were persuaded to adopt the necessary program of vigorous activity, the savings would become ($428 × 0.5 × 0.2), or $42.80 per worker-year. The

Table 2.3 The Influence of Physical Activity Upon Various Indices of Ischemic Heart Disease, Expressed as the Ratio of Incidence for Active and Inactive Populations

Index of Ischemic Heart Disease	Mean Ratio	Range	Number of Studies
Myocardial pain	0.48	0.21-0.68	8
Angina pectoris	1.36	0.65-1.98	7
Myocardial infarction	0.56	0.33-0.98	9
Coronary heart disease			
Attack rate	0.60	0.17-1.03	16
Mortality	0.66	0.28-1.22	21
Vascular pathology	0.76	0.51-1.00	7

Note. Table based on data accumulated by S. Fox and W. Haskell, 1968, and S. Fox and W. Haskell, 1967, Population Studies, *Canadian Medical Association Journal,* **96**, pp. 806-809, and from ''Physical Activity and the Prevention of Coronary Heart Disease'' by S. Fox and D.L. Haskell, 1968, Bulletin of the New York Academy of Sciences, **44**, pp. 950-965.

Table 2.4 Relative Risk of Cardiovascular Disease in Active and Inactive Subjects

Populations Compared	Mean Risk Ratio for Active Group	Principal Author
Bus conductors/drivers	0.53	Morris (1953)
Postal carriers/clerks	0.53-0.71	Kahn (1963)
Rail switchmen/clerks	0.50	Taylor (1962)
Harvard alumni	0.63	Paffenbarger (1978)
Civil servants (leisure > 31.5 kJ $\cdot$ min^{-1})	0.38	Morris (1973)
Longshoremen	0.50	Paffenbarger (1977)
Framingham population	0.40	Kannel (1979)
Health Insurance Plan New York	0.50	Shapiro (1969)
Kibbutzim residents		Brunner (1974)
Male	0.40	
Female	0.32	
Citizens of Oslo	0.33	Holme (1981)

Note. From *The Economic Benefits of Participation in Regular Physical Activity* (p. 7) by A.D. Roberts, 1982, Canberra, Australia: Recreation Ministers' Council of Australia.

Ontario data (Table 2.1) exclude costs attributable to medical education, research, and intangibles. Again, subtracting the allowance for premature death, the total becomes $774M, or $282.50 per worker-year. The expected savings, $28.25 per worker-year, are thus somewhat less than the

Table 2.5 Relative Risk of Fatal Heart Attack in Californian Longshoremen With Low Energy Output

Type of Death	Risk Ratio for Active Group (Work > 21.8 kJ • min^{-1})
Sudden	0.30
Delayed	0.63
Unspecified	0.59
All deaths	0.50

Note. Based on data of R. Paffenbarger, 1977. Data adjusted for age, cigarette consumption, and blood pressure.

Table 2.6 Risk of First Heart Attack in Sedentary Harvard Alumni Relative to Those Taking Voluntary Leisure Activity of at Least 8000 kJ • wk^{-1}

Smoking Habit	Risk Ratio for Active Group
Cigarette smokers	0.45
Nonsmokers	0.65
All subjects	0.63

Note. From "Physical Activity as an Index of Heart Attack Risk in College Alumni" by R. Paffenbarger, A.L. Wing, and R. T. Hyde, 1978, *American Journal of Epidemiology, 108,* pp. 161-175.

U.S. figure. Klarman (1964) included all forms of cardiovascular disease in his estimate, arguing that it was not particularly fruitful to attempt to apportion costs between different diagnoses. In contrast, the Quasar study took the total costs of cardiovascular disease for the Province of Ontario, divided this by the number of cardiovascular "hospital separations," and thus obtained an approximate estimate of cost per incident ($5844) that could be applied to the coronary attack rate. The Quasar calculation assumes that all forms of cardiovascular disease have a similar cost.

Roberts (1982) argued that it was desirable to disaggregate the cardiovascular total into its component bed-days—acute myocardial infarction (21%), other ischemic heart diseases (16%), symptomatic heart disease (23%), and cerebrovascular disease (40%). On this basis, 12% of Australian hospital costs were attributable to the cardiovascular system, but only 7.2% were attributable to the treatment of coronary diseases. The distinction has some importance, less clear because it is that exercise will reduce the costs of cerebrovascular disease. Moreover, Roberts (1982) distinguished a 20-week morbidity period for ischemic heart disease, compared to a 10-week absence from work for symptomatic heart disease, whereas Quasar (1976) allowed a standard 13 weeks of morbidity for all nonfatal episodes.

Among other direct costs, Roberts estimated that 77% of medical consultation expenses, 80% of pharmaceutical purchases, and 56% of ambulance use were attributable to the coronary component of cardiovascular disease. Estimates of the direct costs to the national economy of a single cardiovascular incident were similar to the Ontario data as were all costs of coronary heart disease except the loss of production from premature death (which he estimated at about $176 per worker-year). Nevertheless, scope remains to recalculate costs for Canada and the U.S., using the more precise disaggregated technique proposed by Roberts.

With regard to the other chronic diseases listed in Table 2.2, any benefit of physical activity is indirect through changes in such facets of lifestyle as tobacco addiction and alcohol abuse. Detailed costing of an average cigarette habit (from the viewpoint of an employer) is presented in Table 2.7. The productivity figure, although large, is based on the as-

Table 2.7 Potential Costs to the Employer of a Smoking Employee

Excess insurance costs per average smoker	$401-419
Health	$298
Fire	$ 15
Workmen's compensation and other accidents	$ 58
Life insurance and early disability	$ 30-48
Other annual costs per average smoker	$498
Absenteeism*	$117
Productivity	$242
Involuntary smoking	$139
Total cost	$899-917
Potential short-run (1-3 year) savings from successful withdrawal	
Fire, workmen's compensation, accidents	$ 73
Absenteeism	$117
Productivity	$242
Involuntary smoking	$ 80
Total savings	$512

*On average, smokers are absent about 2 days more per year than nonsmokers due to such problems as the longer duration of upper-respiratory infections.

Note. From "The Economics of Health Promotion at the Work Site" by M. Kristein, 1982, *Health Education Quarterly,* **9** (Suppl.), pp. 27-36.

Costs are converted to 1983 Canadian dollars.

sumption that an equivalent of 8 min of work per day are lost through the smoking ritual, extra clean-up costs, damage (to equipment, furniture, and fixtures), and errors due to eye irritation. Another U.S. estimate found additional costs equivalent to $5.50 per day for each smoking employee; the total burden amounted to 81 million days of work loss and a productivity deficit of $19 billion (Danaher, 1980).

The maximum likely lifestyle benefit from an exercise program is a doubling of successful cigarette withdrawal (Morgan, Gildiner, & Wright, 1976) with a small improvement in the success of alcohol withdrawal (Wilbur, 1983). But an additional complication is that heavy consumers of cigarettes and alcohol are not generally attracted to fitness and lifestyle programs. More data are needed concerning both impact and outcome, but possible assumptions are that (a) 20% of workers and their spouses will adopt a program of vigorous exercise, (b) 20% of this subgroup will initially have had cigarette and/or alcohol addiction, and (c) 50% of those who were initially addicted will have been cured by the program. The effectiveness thus drops to (0.2) (0.2) (0.5) with some 2% of the labor force stopping smoking and/or reducing alcohol consumption.

If 35% of the target population are initially cigarette addicts, the ultimate savings are (2/35)100, or 5.7%, of costs for cigarette-related disorders. About 10% of the target population are likely to have a major alcohol addiction, and if alcohol intake is greatly curtailed in 2% of individuals this could save (2/10)100, or 20%, of alcohol-related costs. Unfortunately, the success rate is likely to be low among those subjects who are the heaviest drinkers. A combined estimate of 5.7% cost savings may be set for both alcohol- and cigarette-related disorders, recognizing that this is a rather crude estimate in need of further refinement.

Self-reports from the Toronto Life Assurance Study (Shephard, Corey, & Cox, 1982—3% smoking withdrawal) and from the Johnson & Johnson Corporation in the U.S. (3.5% smoking withdrawal in one year, Wilbur, 1983) support the general magnitude of the assumed effect on the cigarette habit. Some authors (Fletcher, 1959; Berry & Boland, 1977; Luce & Schweitzer, 1978) suggest that as much as a quarter of U.S. annual health costs of $623B are attributable to cigarette and alcohol abuse. Deducting the costs associated with premature death, we are left with a charge to the U.S. economy of 0.25(416.4B) or $104.1B. However, a major component of both the direct costs and the morbidity associated with cigarette and alcohol abuse ($47.1B) is related to cardiovascular disease. The residual cost of the cigarette/alcohol abuse item to the U.S. economy is thus $57B, or $518 per worker-year. Given a 5.7% program effectiveness, the savings from this response to an exercise program would be $29.53 per worker-year. Arbitrarily ascribing $16.53 to the effects of alcohol (cirrhosis, malnutrition, vehicle accidents) and $13.00 to the noncardiac hazards of smoking (chronic chest disease, various forms of cancer, complications of pregnancy), with the maximization of the smoking withdrawal benefit over the first 10 of 20 residual career years (Rogot & Murray, 1980), the fiscal impact would drop to $16.53 + 0.75($13.00), or $26.28 per worker-year.

The overall economic effect is even more complicated because of reductions of accidental fires and losses of revenue from cigarette and alcohol taxation. Berl and Halpin (1978, December) traced 44% of fire fatalities in the state of Maryland to careless smoking. In the U.S., federal, state, and municipal tobacco taxes now yield the equivalent of Canadian $9.6B per year (Tobacco Tax Council, 1980). If the percentage of smokers drops from 35 to 33%, a 2.5% reduction will occur in the incidence of major fires [(2/35) × 0.44] and tax revenues will decrease by [9.6 × (2/35)] $0.55B per year ($5.00 per worker-year). Some argue that cigarette and alcohol taxes are transfer payments and thus should be excluded from cost-benefit analyses. This is probably correct in terms of the overall economy, but from the governmental perspective, money that is not spent on tobacco or alcohol may be diverted to consumer purchases with a much lower revenue yield (chapter 3).

The basic calculations on the costs of chronic disease may be checked using the data of Table 2.2. Noncardiac items generate direct costs of $735.8M for the Ontario population. Moreover, morbidity costs for noncardiac items ($68.1M) are proportionately 30% higher than for cardiac items. Summing direct and morbidity columns thus gives a total of $803.9M for noncardiac items. Given 5.7% program effectiveness and a working population of 2.74 million, the benefit from this response ($16.72 per worker-year) is of the same general order as observed in the U.S. Allocating $9.37 of the $16.72 to alcohol and $7.35 to smoking effects, and distributing the latter savings over the first 10 of a 20-year residual career span, the Ontario statistics suggest equivalent savings of ($9.37 + $5.51) or $14.88 per worker-year.

Medical and Hospital Costs

Several Russian authors (cited by Dodov, Ploshtakov, Patcharazon, & Nilolova, 1975; and Pravosudov, 1978) have found better levels of health in physically active workers than in those not participating in sport and physical culture. However, the studies appear to be cross-sectional in nature, with no quantitation of the amounts of activity undertaken by sport enthusiasts and sedentary groups.

Likewise, a cross-sectional analysis of Ontario Health Insurance Plan payments (Quasar, 1976) suggested that costs to the plan would be reduced by 5.5% if all adults aged 20-69 years had at least an average level of cardiorespiratory fitness. From the prevalence of cardiac risk factors in the adult population of Ontario, it was further estimated that if everyone was brought to an adequate level of fitness, future ischemic heart disease costs would decrease by the current equivalent of $29M per year (Quasar, 1976; Megalli, 1978, May). Two flaws in this reasoning are that (a) nothing guarantees that an increase of personal fitness would correct all risk factors (although often some improvement of risk profile is apparent as activity is enhanced), and (b) nothing guarantees that the removal of a risk factor late in adult life would avert a subsequent cardiac incident.

Knezevich (1980) noted that a 17-week employee fitness program at Ontario Hydro's head office decreased body fat, serum cholesterol, and blood pressure. He estimated that those who completed the program reduced their 5-year heart attack risks by 36.5% and their 20-year risks by 33.4%. In this company 44.6% of all employee deaths and 20% of all absenteeism were attributable to diseases of the heart and circulatory system.

Corrigan (1980) examined nonaccidental health insurance claims at Purdue University (West Lafayette, IN). The frequency of claims was similar for 29 continuing participants and 15 dropouts from the University's adult fitness program. Continuing participants had significantly lower total dollar claims than dropouts (equivalent to charges of $54.40 per year for the exercisers, compared to $106.52 in controls, saving $52.10 per exerciser per year). However, excluding the possibility that initial differences of health or personality may have been responsible for defections from the fitness program is difficult. A similar criticism can be made of data from the "Staywell" program of U.S. Control Data Corporation, which showed 36% higher health-care costs and 54% longer hospital stays among employees who did not exercise.

Shephard et al. (1981) obtained self-reports of illness from participants in the Toronto Life Assurance study. Their findings showed that after introduction of a fitness/lifestyle program at one of two similar companies, employees at the experimental company made fewer visits to the industrial nurse or physician, spent less time in the hospital, and purchased fewer prescription drugs than the sedentary controls. Moreover, when experimental subjects were subdivided on the basis of their program adherence, high adherents reported the largest reduction in colds and absenteeism. Nevertheless, both willingness to complete questionnaires and program adherence were factors of self-selection. Although the results were encouraging, it was thus difficult to draw firm economic conclusions from these preliminary findings.

Shephard, Corey, Renzland, and Cox (1982) were able to obtain somewhat more satisfactory proof of employee fitness program benefits through a longitudinal examination of grouped Ontario Health Insurance

Plan (OHIP) records for the same two companies. Their calculations were based on claims submitted to the Provincial medical insurance scheme (OHIP) over 2 successive years (1977 and 1978). An employee fitness program was initiated at the experimental company in January 1978. Linkage between experimental data and OHIP records was based upon concordance of three identifiers (health insurance number, age, and sex) and thus allowed for situations in which two members of a family had used the same OHIP number or an alteration of marital status had given one claimant two OHIP numbers. It proved necessary to delete 2.3% of the subjects due to difficulty in establishing unequivocal data linkage. Of the subjects who were accepted for statistical analysis, 5.5% had no medical or hospital claims, 82.4% had medical claims only, and 12.1% had both medical and hospital claims. At the control company, hospital bed usage increased from 0.13 days per employee-year in 1977 to 0.51 days per employee-year in 1978, whereas at the experimental company a drop occurred from 0.27 to 0.09 days per employee-year (Table 2.8). Because of rounding, the true gain from the program ($P < 0.02$) was 0.57 days per employee-year. Nonparticipants in the fitness/lifestyle program had higher initial hospital utilizations than participants, but both categories of employees (participants and nonparticipants) contributed to the healthcare savings at the experimental company.

Medical claims were grouped into five categories—total claims, electrocardiography, orthopedic services, obstetric and gynecological services, and other services. Total claims increased at the control company from 1977 to 1978, due in part to an increase in the approved medical fee schedule (Table 2.8). In contrast, the potential increase of claims was largely contained at the experimental company. The net savings on medical claims attributable to the fitness/lifestyle program thus amounted to $45.40 per employee-year (approximately equivalent to three medical consultations).

Table 2.8 Saving in OHIP Claims With Introduction of Fitness/Lifestyle Program at Company A (1978)*

Claims	Company A		Company B		Net Saving
	1977	1978	1977	1978	
Hospital bed-days ($ per employee-year)	43.20	14.39	27.18	81.55	83.18
Medical costs ($ per employee-year)	134.63	135.92	135.12	181.81	45.40
					$128.58

*Company B served as control throughout. Hospital beds cost $160/day (1983 dollars).

Table 2.9 Changes in OHIP Claims for Electrocardiographic and Orthopedic Services With Introduction of Fitness/Lifestyle Program at Company A (1978)*

Services	Company A 1977	Company A 1978	Company B 1977	Company B 1978	Net Saving
ECG services ($)	0.27	0.40	0.30	0.32	−0.11
Orthopedic services ($)	3.20	3.90	3.63	6.20	1.87
					1.76

*Company B served as control throughout (1983 dollars).

Again, the savings were shown rather equally by all employees at the experimental company, whether they were participants or nonparticipants in the fitness/lifestyle program. It was anticipated that participation in the exercise classes might have generated substantial extra costs for electrocardiographic and orthopedic services, but this did not prove to be the case (Table 2.9).

The total savings in health-care costs at the experimental company amounted to $128.58 per employee-year when expressed in 1983 Canadian currency. Several comments on this statistic follow:

(a) No allowance has been made for possible administrative savings. Operating costs of OHIP (salaries, supplies, technical services, and computing) add about 5% to the bills submitted for medical consultations and hospital care, while utilization of governmental office space adds a further 1-2%. However, nothing guarantees that the 6-7% surcharge on physician and hospital payments could be recovered, particularly if physical activity reduced the size rather than the total number of OHIP billings.

(b) Savings on hospital care as a result of an increase in population fitness could only be realized if the total number of beds were reduced or new construction previously planned for an aging population was avoided.

(c) Health-care costs are an outcome measure. However, the period of observation was insufficient to observe some of the more important outcomes, including any possible reduction of chronic disease—the savings observed in the first year of the experiment must have resulted from either a lower incidence of acute disease or (more probably) from a reduction in consultations for complaints that lacked any firm organic basis. A longer-term study might well reveal much larger health-care savings.

(d) Because all categories of workers at the experimental company benefited from the fitness program, the data suggest that the reduced OHIP costs reflected a general increase of employee life-satisfaction or a diffusion of health education propaganda throughout the company, rather than a more specific effect of the fitness program upon disease. Support for this last assumption is found in relatively limited coefficients of correlation between changes of health-care costs and changes of physical fitness or health hazard appraisal scores (Shephard, Corey, & Cox, 1982).

Because the period of observation was short, a need exists to check whether the reduction in costs was maintained. Observations also need to be repeated on a much larger population. Medical benefits were at the borderline of formal statistical significance, and the major item in the calculation (reduced hospital bed-days) could reflect mainly the experience of a small number of individuals admitted for treatment of chronic diseases. In particular, the 0.38-day per worker-year *increase* of hospital usage by employees at the control company seems likely to be an artifact of sample size.

Because the overall balance sheet includes no other entry for the costs of acute medical care in adults, the estimated medical and hospital-care savings should be added to the tally of personal benefits derived from a fitness/lifestyle program. Possibly because a total environmental change occurred at the experimental company, the impact upon OHIP costs seen by Shephard, Corey, Renzland, and Cox (1982) was larger than would have been predicted from the Quasar study. The Toronto Life Assurance data is in closer agreement with the insurance billings of Corrigan (1980) and the results of the Staywell program, although such comparisons are complicated by higher medical charges in the U.S.

Rehabilitation

A suitable graded exercise plan speeds recovery from many illnesses, allows a faster return to normal work, and reduces the risk of recurrence of disability. However, the necessary programs are specialized, quite costly, and fall outside the scope of the present analysis.

Of more interest is the potential facilitation of rehabilitation by prior physical activity. For example, Weinblatt et al. (1966) suggested that a history of prior vigorous physical activity doubled the chances of return to full-time work following myocardial infarction. Scope is available for a more detailed analysis of the potential savings, although Weinblatt may have overstated the benefit of prior exercise, because recent reports show an 85-88% return to work with post hoc rehabilitation irrespective of previous activity habits. Moreover, age, motivation, skills, experience, financial status, and attitudes of relatives all have a major impact upon the likelihood of a return to normal employment following a major illness (Shephard, 1981). Reference to Table 2.1 illustrates the order of importance of the rehabilitation item. The Quasar calculation allowed postcoronary patients an average of 3 months convalescence following an infarction, at a cost of $45M ($16.40 per worker-year). However, the 12% of postcoronary patients who fail to return to work would rob society of a 40-80 times larger per capita sum (10-20 years of lost production, at a potential cost of at least $45 × 40 × 12/100, or $216M, $79 per worker-year). Accepting the assertion of Weinblatt et al. (1966), that prior exercise halves the number of persistently unemployed patients, then the savings associated with 20% participation in an exercise program would amount to $7.90 per worker-year. Conceivably, this figure should be augmented if (as is likely) regular physical activity facilitates the recovery from conditions other than coronary vascular disease.

Nutrition

The main nutritional consequences of enhanced physical activity are an increased energy intake, a reduction of body fat, and an improved blood lipid profile.

Energy Intake

The body can store only limited amounts of energy, so the long-term consequence of vigorous physical activity must be an increased intake of food. Suppose an average middle-aged person with a maximum oxygen intake of $2.2 \, l \cdot min^{-1}$ exercises according to the recommended training schedule (five 30-min sessions per week at 60% of maximum oxygen intake). The rate of energy expenditure will be $27.6 \, kJ \cdot min^{-1}$ ($6.6 \, kcal \cdot min^{-1}$), which is an increase over sedentary rest of $20.9 \, kJ \cdot min^{-1}$ ($5.0 \, kcal \cdot min^{-1}$). The added energy demand will then amount to $31.4 \, MJ \cdot wk^{-1}$, or $750 \, kcal \cdot wk$, a 4.3% increase of food consumption. Given an annual food consumption of $1000 per head and 20% participation of the adult population in an exercise program, the added food bill would be about $15.80 per worker-year. The fluid loss from sweating (about 0.5 liters per exercise session) is probably insufficient to modify beverage consumption, although more vigorous and protracted activity (such as a "fun run") could generate a demand for 3-4 liters of replacement fluids.

Vitamin Intake

Nutrition experts have long known that the individual who is vulnerable to vitamin deficiencies (Durnin, 1973) combines a low total energy intake with ingestion of a substantial proportion of empty calories (refined carbohydrates and alcohol). Conversely, the active individual who eats a well-balanced diet is unlikely to need vitamin supplements. A physical activity program thus reduces the need for expensive synthetic vitamin preparations.

In practice, active individuals probably will not realize any savings without extensive health education. On the contrary, those who choose to exercise commonly consume an above average proportion of vitamin preparations (Kavanagh & Shephard, 1977).

Reduction of Body Fat

Physical activity is a pleasant and effective long-term method of correcting moderate obesity (Sidney, Shephard, & Harrison, 1977; Kukkonen et al., 1982b). Exercise has many advantages over alternative types of therapy. Mood is elevated, some suppression of appetite is possible, lean tissue loss is avoided, and the risk of inducing ventricular fibrillation is less than with severe dieting. Above all, the patient learns a new lifestyle and is less likely to fall back into former bad habits.

Many of the fiscal benefits arising from a correction of obesity have already been noted under chronic illness. However, savings may come from a lesser consumption of food or snacks as fat is being metabolized. Suppose that 10 kg of fat are burned. This provides 293 megajoules (MJ) of energy (70,000 kcal), which equals food needs for about 27 days. The bonus occurs once only. This bonus is worth perhaps $74 per individual with a wise choice of food purchases, but as much as $3000 if distributed over expensive snacks (Rhodes, 1982, May). Distributed over a lifetime, with 20% participation, the annual benefit ranges from $1 to $40 per person, or $0.50-$20 per worker-year.

The reduction of body mass might cause a sustained decrease in the discretionary (active) component of the total energy expenditure (4.18 MJ, 1000 kcal per day). The effect would be roughly proportional to the change of body mass, so that a drop from 75 to 65 kg could reduce discretionary expenditures by 13% and overall expenditures by 5.2%. If the savings were realized, with 20% program participation the yield would be $19.10 per worker-year. Scope is available for further study of food needs after slimming. However, it seems quite likely that the rejuvenated individual will become more active and will dissipate much of the potential financial advantage from any reduction of body mass. Nevertheless, this item could well be sufficient to offset the additional food needs suggested for participation in a training program.

Lipid Profile

If a certain threshold intensity of training is surpassed, regular exercise induces favorable changes in the lipid profile, particularly increasing the level of the scavenger "HDL cholesterol" (Medalie, Tyroler, & Heiss, 1980). Also, such changes are likely to reduce the risk of subsequent coronary vascular disease. Fiscal allowance for this item has already been made under *chronic diseases*.

Changes of Lifestyle

Becoming involved in a regular physical activity program without developing a positive attitude toward health is difficult. Class leaders, peers, and promotional booklets all encourage positive health, and many program participants are encouraged to stop smoking, reduce their alcohol consumptions, and adopt more prudent lifestyles. Body mass and serum cholesterol levels fall, and an appreciable reduction of systemic blood pressures occurs. Such a clustering of good health habits and their practical outcomes has been discussed by Hickey, Mulcahy, Bourke, Graham, and Wilson-Davis (1975), Cooper, Pollock, Martin, White, Linnerud, and Jackson (1976), Breslow and Enstrom (1980), and Erikssen, Forfang, and Jervell (1981). Santa Barbara (1982b) further argues that the increase of physical activity usually precedes other improvements of lifestyle.

The impact of improved lifestyle upon morbidity and direct health-care costs has already been considered under *chronic illnesses*. However, useful savings are also available from a reduction in premature mortality. Breslow and Enstrom (1980) found that in active men the 9-1/2-year age-adjusted mortality rate was only 36.5% of that for sedentary individuals, while in active women the rate was 40.4% of the sedentary figure. The net impact of improved lifestyle has been examined using the Health Hazard Appraisal technique (Shephard, Corey, & Cox, 1982). The Health Hazard Appraisal instrument calculates a composite risk score for any given individual, along with a corresponding appraised age. Cross-sectional studies show that the composite risk score is negatively correlated with maximum oxygen intake and muscular vigor (Landry, LeBlanc, Gaudreau, & Moisan, 1982). If the individual's risk-taking behavior remains unchanged over a longitudinal study, then the appraised age should increase parallel to the calendar age. Thus in the Toronto Life

Table 2.10 Change of Appraised Age With 6 Months of Participation in Employee Fitness Program

Subject Category	Change of Appraised Age	Percent of Sample	Gain of Appraised Age
Control subjects	+0.48 years	100	0.02 years
Experimental subjects			
Nonparticipants	+1.07 years	50	-1.57 years
Dropouts	-0.26 years	10	0.76 years
Low-adherents	+0.05 years	20	0.45 years
High-adherents	-0.76 years	20	1.26 years

Note. From "Health Hasard Appraisal—The Influence of an Employee Fitness Programme" by R.J. Shephard, P. Corey, and M. Cox, 1982, *Canadian Journal of Public Health*, **73**, pp. 183-187.

Assurance study (Table 2.10), control subjects showed almost the expected increase of appraised age when retested after an interval of 6 months (gain of 0.48 years). Nonparticipants in the employee fitness program apparently had some additional deterioration of appraised age relative to the calendar changes of 0.5 years. But dropouts, low adherents, and high adherents to the exercise program all showed less than the expected increase of appraised age. For the purpose of these calculations, all person-years of benefit are attributed to the 20% of the population that became vigorous exercisers. The weighted effect is then a 2.09-year decrease of appraised age.

The ascribed savings depend upon income ($14,500 per year is assumed here), the method of calculation (the conservative index of added value, rather than total earnings, will be used; see chapter 1), and the age of retirement. The benefit is ($14,500 × 0.25 × 2.09 × 0.2), or $1515 per worker assuming that an exerciser who is effectively 2 years younger will work about 2 years longer. Distributed over a working career of 40 years, this item amounts to $37.90 per worker-year. However, if most workers are subjected to compulsory retirement, the benefit is applicable only to the 20% of the population that would otherwise have died between the ages of 25 and 65 years. The savings then drop to $7.58 per worker-year. Neither of these calculations makes any allowance for the personal value of survival into retirement, nor has any figure yet been introduced for the services of full-time homemakers. If 10% of the labor force keep house at a value of $7250 per year, the above figures must be increased by 5% to $39.80 and $7.96 per worker-year respectively.

Learning Processes

Persuading adults to become physically more active is difficult. The ideal time for developing the habit of regular physical activity is thus during the years of attendance at primary school. However, the argument is sometimes advanced that curricular time cannot be spared for required physical activity—the opportunity cost is too great with respect to the demands of the academic curriculum.

Volle, Shephard et al. (1982) examined this issue in a study of primary school students (see Table 2.11). They demonstrated that, far from impairing the learning process, the addition of 1 hr per day of physical activity to the curriculum enhanced learning, possibly through an acceleration of psychomotor development (Volle, Tisal et al., 1982).

The ultimate value of the enhanced academic learning is hard to quantify, particularly if the effect of exercise is mainly to speed the learning process. As the children involved in this study mature, it may become possible to compare the average incomes of those originally assigned to experimental and control groups. The only negative effect of the program observed to date has been a small increase of absenteeism in Grade 1. The cost of this has already been noted.

Programs for young children are generally considered the responsibility of the school board or the municipality, but in the U.S., a Junior Gym is selling eight "rhythmic experiences" for the equivalent of $69.

Table 2.11 The Influence of 5 Hours Per Week of Required Physical Education Upon the Academic Standing of Primary School Students

Academic Grade (Averaged Over Subjects)	Rural Milieu		Urban Milieu	
	Experimental %	Control %	Experimental %	Control %
A	65.5	52.2	42.8	38.6
B	23.8	33.0	41.2	39.3
C	7.8	10.8	15.1	16.5
D, E, or F	2.9	4.1	0.9	5.6

$P < 0.001$.

Note. From "Influence of a Programme of Required Physical Activity Upon Academic Performance" by M. Volle, R.J. Shephard, H. Lavallée, R. LaBarre, J.C. Jéquier, and M. Rajic, 1982, in H. Lavallée and R.J. Shephard (Eds.), *Croissance et Développement de l'Enfant* (p. 95), Trois Rivières: University of Québec at Trois Rivières.

In 1981, gross revenues of the Junior Gym operation equaled $320,000, with a profit of $126,000 (Reed, 1981, November 2).

Conclusions

The cost-benefit ledger for the personal consequences of physical activity is summarized in Table 2.12. But on the credit side of the ledger, information that would enable us to assign any precise value to a variety of opportunity dividends is lacking. The largest measured items are acute hospital and medical costs, plus a decrease in premature mortality. The

Table 2.12 Balance Sheet for Personal Consequences of Enhanced Physical Activity*

Credit		Debit	
Opportunity dividends	$?	Opportunity cost	25-50 hours
(Physical stamina		Child-care, Grade I	$ 7.70[a]
Appearance		Decreased revenues[b]	
Heat tolerance		Cigarettes	($ 5.00)
Protection against injuries		Alcohol	($?)
Flexibility		Increased food consumption	$15.80
Improved mood)			$28.50
Cardiovascular disease			
(Direct costs + morbidity)	$ 28.25		
Other disease			
(Direct costs + morbidity)	$ 14.88		
Reduced fire hazards	$?		
Acute hospital and medical costs	$128.59		
Rehabilitation			
Postcoronary	$ 7.90		
Other diseases	$?		
Decreased vitamin needs	$?		
Fat usage	$ 0.50		
Decreased body mass	$ 19.10		
Reduced premature mortality	$ 39.80[†]		
Enhanced academic learning	$?		
	$239.02		

*All costs are shown per worker-year assuming 20% participation in the exercise program.

[a]100% participation assumed for this item.

[b]Some authors would argue that these are transfer payments and thus should be excluded from a cost-benefit analysis.

[†]$7.96 if retirement age not adjusted.

magnitude of benefit attributable to this last item depends upon legislation governing mandatory retirement (at present in a state of flux). Other benefits that currently lack accurate fiscal estimates are reduced fire hazards, a speeding of rehabilitation from diseases other than heart attacks, a decreased need for synthetic vitamins, and an enhancement of academic learning.

On the debit side, the opportunity cost of exercise (250-300 hrs per year) is substantial, even if charged at the minimum wage. However, many observers would make the value judgment that opportunity costs are fully offset by the opportunity dividends of exercise. Another debatable item is whether "lost" tobacco and alcohol revenues should be included in the balance sheet. Most economists exclude transfer payments from their calculations, although the money "saved" through a reduction of tobacco purchases could well move from government to private coffers.

If due allowance were made for the unmeasured credits, the personal balance sheet would probably show a substantial margin in favor of enhanced physical activity.

chapter 3

Sociocultural Considerations

The level of sports finance is a key factor affecting participation in sport. (Rodgers, 1978)

Many of the limitations of the existing data on leisure spending arise because there is neither an agreed definition of leisure nor a sufficient concern with an overall concept of leisure. As a result, official statisticians have had no real incentive either to attempt to produce figures relating to aggregate leisure spending or to overcome some of the real problems of measurement that leisure poses. (Martin and Mason, 1983, p. 43)

Enlightened company physicians have sometimes questioned the need to provide an economic justification for employee fitness and health programs (Jacobs & Chovil, 1983), arguing that a medical department is hardly set up with a view to earning profits. The same type of reasoning can be espoused by national governments—good health and personal fitness are fringe benefits of living in a well-ordered society and do not require justification on a cost-benefit scale. Like many other fringe benefits, fitness probably has some favorable influence upon national economic activity, but much of the effect may be too circuitous to allow direct measurement (Alchian & Kessel, 1977; Atherley et al., 1976). Lack of cost-benefit statistics should not become an excuse for rejecting programs.

While any national government might well subscribe to such altruism and indeed would wish the financial resources to tackle all social problems simultaneously, in practice a finite capacity exists both to initiate and to sustain programs. As fitness and lifestyle promotion and programs mature, they therefore come under close scrutiny for process, impact, and outcome (chapter 1). Potential advantages of physical activity must be weighed carefully against other social priorities, and the ultimate criterion should be a cost-benefit analysis. The fiscal impact of fitness programing cannot be considered in isolation, for any increase of physical activity has profound implications for other sectors of the economy, including such components as tourism, spectator sports, passive entertainment, and cigarette and beer manufacturing. Moreover, the likelihood of involvement in many forms of physical activity is strongly dependent upon the socioeconomic status of the individual. The present chapter will examine some of these sociocultural issues.

Social Priorities for the Government

The balance sheet presented in chapter 7 suggests that exercise may have a beneficial effect not only upon personal and corporate health, but also upon the national exchequer. Nevertheless, before embarking upon heavy investment in exercise programing, the government must consider the following:

1. The issue of personal versus societal responsibility
2. The effectiveness of exercise relative to alternative types of personal health programing
3. The acceptability of physical activity promotion
4. The relative ease with which various types of behavioral change can be promoted and induced

Personal Versus Societal Responsibility

When dealing with any health problem, apportioning responsibility between personal behavior and nonbehavioral influences is important (McGinnis, 1981; Green, Kreuter, Deeds, & Portridge, 1980; Allison & Coburn, 1981; Godin & Shephard, in press). Some social historians have argued that the physical inactivity of the modern apartment-dweller is not a personal failing, but is rather a reflection of present urban conditions. A sedentary lifestyle has been induced by the migration to large cities, where there is inadequate open space and little opportunity to pursue traditional rural pastimes. Structural changes in North American society have led to a substitution of spectator sport for personal activity (Redlich, 1965; Ingham & Beamish, 1983); this process has been fostered by such interests as streetcar and railway companies (Betts, 1974), newspapers (Cozens & Stumpf, 1953), and most recently commercial television stations (Clement, 1975). A logical deduction from such arguments is that the inactive individual should not be criticized for a lack of personal responsibility. Blame for adverse health behavior should be directed rather to his or her cultural environment (R.F. Allen, 1977; Duare & Kreuter, 1981; Pellegrino, 1981; Veatch, 1982).

Some self-styled Critical Theorists imply further that the cultural impediment to a desirable level of habitual activity would be removed in a Marxist Utopia. In fact, no good evidence exists to show that present forms of state socialism engender a healthy lifestyle; television watching is the dominant leisure pursuit in East as in West Germany (Stundl, 1977) and the percentage of regular sports participants is remarkably similar on both sides of the iron curtain (Stundl, 1977; Bischoff & Maldaner, 1980). Nevertheless, when seeking fitness recruits, one should look critically at the cost-effectiveness of an overall improvement of socioeconomic conditions and cultural change relative to the merits of more personal fitness propaganda.

The traditional North American viewpoint of health as a personal responsibility (Hofstadter, 1955) is still echoed by many Protestant fundamentalists. If their stance is correct, it becomes quite logical to encourage fitness through such mechanisms as vigorous advertising and differential health premiums that favor those attaining desirable standards of physical condition.

As with most arguments, some truth is present in the positions held by extremists of both camps. Current psychological models (Fishbein & Ajzen, 1974; Godin & Shephard, in press, 1986) stress the major impact of both environment and societal norms upon health behavior. Too often, the external structural constraints postulated by the Critical Theorists do play a role in keeping the individual from a desirable lifestyle (Wikler, 1978; Tsalikis, 1980; Labonté & Penfold, 1981). Thus urban conditions can and should be modified to encourage the activities of pedestrians and cyclists (chapter 6).

Society can and should moderate its enthusiasm for spectator events and high-cost leisure and should encourage in their stead enjoyable low-cost pursuits that can be enjoyed by families with slender margins of disposable income. On the other hand, given that most people will continue in sedentary employment and many will also live in large apartment complexes, environmental change unlikely can go more than halfway toward encouraging personal physical activity. Ultimately, the individual must also assume some responsibility and make a deliberate decision to undertake sufficient exercise to maintain his or her health. The government also should be directing at least a part of its efforts to securing such a personal commitment.

Effectiveness

The main obstacle in assessing the health benefits of exercise is the impossiblity of persuading large and representative samples of the general population to participate in any type of extended, randomized, controlled trial. Inferences concerning the value of exercise must therefore be drawn from epidemiological comparisons of subjects differing in their self-selected patterns of physical activity. Note in passing that the problem is not peculiar to the assessment of fitness programs. Allocating the general population randomly to regimens that require a high cigarette consumption, a low fat intake, or an administration of hypotensive drugs over an extended period is equally impossible.

The most clear-cut long-term measure of health outcome is the total mortality of a population. Paffenbarger (1977) concluded that on this criterion an increase of physical activity was at least as effective in reducing mortality as was a reduction of systemic blood pressure or cigarette consumption. Others have noted that heavy cigarette smoking (> 40 cigarettes/day) reduces the life expectancy of a 25-year-old man by 8 years, and in this context the 2 year gain of appraised age developed by a person who becomes more active (chapter 2) seems to be a less dramatic reward. On the other hand, the physiological gains associated with regular physical activity may well be equivalent to an 8-9 year reduction of physiological age (chapter 5), a benefit at least as large as that suggested for cigarette withdrawal. Another important argument (chapter 2) is that an increase of physical activity has a favorable impact upon possible alternative foci of intervention such as smoking, obesity, and hypertension.

On present evidence, it may be concluded that the promotion of physical activity is likely to have as much benefit as any other unimodal tactic of health promotion, with the possible exception of the encouragement of smoking cessation. Not only are the benefits large, but cost-effectiveness is quite good for a smoking withdrawal clinic; if success is achieved, the expense is of a once-only nature, whereas an exercise program requires continuing investment (chapter 7).

The relative merits of fitness promotion and environmental change are less clearly established. For example, in a hot and noisy factory, outcome might be evaluated in terms of labor turnover and productivity. In such a situation, it seems possible that the most cost-effective method of reducing turnover and improving productivity might be to control the noise at the source and to install air conditioning; a noontime fitness class would prove to be a poor substitute for such environmental control. However, it is interesting that in the deep mines of South Africa (where air conditioning costs are very high) preliminary physical conditioning of miners has been a useful tactic. A second common problem limiting corporate performance is poor decision-making on the part of an overstressed executive; in such a situation, the cost-effectiveness of exercise, yoga, and progressive relaxation as stress-reducing techniques is fairly easy to compare, but costing environmental approaches to the control of stress is more difficult.

It has sometimes been argued that both government and industry could sidestep difficult decisions on the effectiveness of exercise versus other types of lifestyle modification or a more general environmental change through the introduction of a "quality of life" package. But even if funding is available for such a Utopian solution, the careful planner must apportion the available budget between the various elements of such a package.

Acceptability

Most health promotional tactics have negative connotations—the public is urged to eat less, give up eggs and rich meat, stop smoking, avoid drinking alcohol, and reduce the variety or frequency of sexual intercourse. Physical activity has the immediate attraction of being one of the few positive actions that can be taken to improve health. Moreover, physical activity is generally regarded as enjoyable. While self-reports must be viewed with some skepticism, the majority of participants in an exercise class will volunteer the information that it makes them feel better, and this accords with the psychophysiological concept of arousal. Unless demands upon the subject are excessive, an improvement of body image can be demonstrated by objective psychological tests (Shephard, 1978), and given progression to vigorous training there may also be a production of mood-elevating hormones (endorphins).

Such personal rewards (opportunity dividends) encourage acceptance of exercise by the general public, with a progression from external motivation (where exercise compliance is poor) to internal motivation (where compliance ranges from good to fanatical). Nevertheless, scope is available to upgrade psychosocial and physical environments, both for the physical activity program itself and for subsequent changing and showering (chapter 6). A surprisingly large proportion of the general public still prefers the pleasure of a weight watchers clinic or a course of hypotensive drugs to the joys of a 2-week canoe voyage through the wilderness. Yet the only negative features threatening the acceptability of physical activity are musculoskeletal injuries (avoided by a gradual progression of training) and the opportunity costs necessary to reach a pleasant exercise environment away from the confines of a large city.

Compliance

As already noted in chapter 2, a final consideration in choice of tactics is the ease with which a given behavior can be induced and sustained (Green et al., 1980). As with other forms of behavioral modification, the main obstacles to promoting an increase of vigorous physical activity are

(a) a limited initial volunteer rate (no more than 40-55% when white-collar workers are offered an in-house program, probably less in a blue-collar or general community setting) and (b) a substantial dropout rate (up to 50% of initial volunteers over the first 6 months of participation in a newly established exercise program).

How may participation rates be improved? The United Steel Corporation in Johannesburg, PA gave a wage increase to employees passing a fitness test (Duggar & Swengros, 1969). Some U.S. companies (Bonnie Belle, Hospital Corporation of America, Forbes Magazine) have attempted to boost participation in employee fitness programs by paying participants or allowing up to 3 hrs of exercise class attendance during the work week (Andrevsky, 1982, December). Nevertheless, the steady attendance rate in most of these programs is still no more than 20%. In the People's Republic of China, the appeal is to party loyalty—as the secretary of one party unit described the fitness break at a Peking auto factory, "It is not a question of whether one finds it (running on a track) interesting or not . . . when one understands the need to keep fit for the revolution, then one should consciously go in for physical training" (Willee, 1976, December, p. 26).

Scope is available (a) to compare compliance rates for exercise and other forms of health intervention using subsets of the same population and (b) to develop tactics for improving all forms of health behavior. Available information suggests that while exercise compliance is not particularly good, it parallels that for most other forms of health promotion. The 1-year success rate for North American smoking withdrawal programs is typically less than 30% (Delarue, 1973), while the long-term success rate of weight reduction is often under 25% (Innes, Campbell, Campbell, Needle, & Munroe, 1974). A Swedish report suggested that 80% of middle-aged men were prepared to take hypotensive drugs for 2 years (Åberg & Hedstrand, 1976), but the sample was small and unrepresentative of the general population. Others have noted quite low rates of compliance with hypotensive therapy in a North American setting. Roberts and Maurer (1977) found that less than one third of U.S. patients with hypertension were taking any form of medication.

Aging modifies both the nature and the extent of participation in physical activity (Nojima, 1978). This has important implications for the cost of both facilities and programs and modifies the effectiveness of exercise promotion (Table 3.1). At present, participation drops sharply once a student leaves school (Canada Fitness Survey, 1983); the late teen years thus seem the most appropriate target for programs designed to sustain active behavior patterns. Attendance at spectator sport events also declines sharply after a student has left school (McPherson & Kozlik, 1980), suggesting that the usual excuse for inactivity (lack of time) may contain a

Table 3.1 Influence of Age Upon Participation in Selected Activities

Age (Years)	Exercise (At Least Once Per Month)	Jog (At Least Once Per Month)	Sport (At Least Once Per Year)	Golf (At Least Once Per Year)	Swim (At Least Once Per Year)
15-16	86.9	53.4	82.0	16.9	60.5
17-19	75.4	34.6	73.3	15.3	53.3
20-24	63.4	19.9	66.3	15.0	44.7
25-34	62.3	12.2	61.3	12.9	38.4
35-44	53.3	9.2	51.2	11.1	30.7
45-54	50.1	5.3	37.2	8.9	20.4
55-64	45.7	2.4	24.5	6.7	11.7
65+	37.0	4.0	9.7	2.5	3.6

Note. From *Culture Statistics—Recreational Activities* (pp. 1-94) by Statistics Canada, 1976, Occasional paper 87-501, Ottawa: Statistics Canada.

germ of truth. On the other hand, television watching shows little decrease over the adult span (McPherson & Kozlik, 1980), and this habit undoubtedly provides a large reservoir of passively occupied leisure time that an individual could allocate to more active pursuits.

Because aging data is largely cross-sectional, interpretation is necessarily speculative. The older individual shows a decreased participation in sport with less frequent attendance as a spectator, and most authors regard these changes as expressions of social disengagement (Atchley, 1977). Physical activity is certainly correlated quite closely with involvement in social networks (Berkman & Syme, 1979), although the lack of activity in the elderly could also be explained if different age cohorts had undergone different socialization experiences. This is an important issue to resolve by further research, for if the older generation has been conditioned to accept long hours of work with little leisure activity as an appropriate lifestyle, it may prove very costly to attempt re-educating them.

An additional explanation is that people have been conditioned to play different roles at different ages. As they become older, priorities may change—partly as a matter of individual choice and partly because of altered structural demands (promotion to a job with lesser physical demands, children leaving home, retirement from work). In general, society expects an older person to slow down and devote time to passive pursuits around the home (Riley, Johnson, & Foner, 1972). If this hypothesis is correct, the main onslaught of geriatric health promoters should be upon structural constraints and inappropriate norms of behavior. A need may also exist to examine marketing techniques. Possibly the leisure industry has directed too much of its advertising to the slim and overtly healthy young adult at the expense of less photogenic middle-aged and older individuals.

Elderly subjects are particularly vulnerable to the opportunity cost of reaching distant facilities. Taylor (1978) discusses some highly cost-effective methods of using small spaces to deliver outdoor activity to the immediate areas where the elderly live.

Socioeconomic Implications of Physical Activity

The fitness and recreation industries, like other areas of leisure spending, are volatile indicators of market conditions. Nevertheless, fluctuations in this sector of the economy have been overlaid by a remarkable growth during the past 2 decades. As early as 1968, the brokerage firm of Merrill Lynch set the U.S. leisure market at an annual figure equivalent to $517 billion; moreover, it was suggested this would grow to $862 billion by 1980 (Merrill Lynch, 1968). In the Province of Ontario, ice hockey and figure skating alone create direct public and private expenditures of $533 million ($75 per citizen), including such items as skate sharpening ($3M), costumes ($8M), ice time, travel, accommodations, and "fast food" (Berger, 1983).

The respective contributions of disposable income and the fitness movement to the growth and recent plateauing of the leisure market will now be examined. Where possible, the implications of leisure patterns for other sectors of the market place will also be explored.

Growth of Active Leisure

Some difficulty exists in establishing secular trends of participation in various forms of physical activity. That is because the basis of data reporting has been inconsistent from year to year, and the standards demanded for an "active" classification in some North American surveys (participation once per month, or even once per year) have been very low relative to those required for a similar classification in Europe (Kuhl, Koch-Nielsen, & Westergaard, 1966; Stundl, 1977). Thomas (1979) suggested that the U.S. at that time had between 10 and 23 million joggers, 15 million serious swimmers, 15 million regular cyclists, and 29 million tennis players. Nevertheless, Breslow and Enstrom (1980) saw no increase in the number of really active adults when data from Alameda County, CA, was compared for the years 1965 and 1974.

The most recent Canadian figures on participation include preliminary information from the Canada Fitness Survey (1983), Fitness Ontario (published report 1981; preliminary unpublished data 1983), Ontario Ministry of Tourism and Recreation (1983), Ferland (1980, November), and Statistics Canada (1975, 1979b, 1980, and 1981). About 77% of able-bodied people participated in one or more sports during 1981, compared with just over 50% in 1976 and 35% in 1972 (Culture Statistics, 1978). Likewise, 66% engaged in active exercise over the preceding month, compared with 63% in 1976 (*exercise* here included such pursuits as walking, jogging, running, cycling, and participating in calisthenics and fitness classes, in contrast to more traditional individual, dual, team, aquatic, and winter sports). Figures for the Province of Ontario were a little lower, with 56-58% noting activity at least once per month in 1979 and 62-70% noting it in 1981.

By way of comparison, in 1972 the Print Measurement Bureau (Conference Board, 1972) carried out a probability sampling of 8000 households, asking subjects over the age of 12 years what activities they did "quite a bit." At this time, only 37% reported sport participation, although 46% worked in the garden and 48% were busy with home improvements. The various statistics suggest that while North America has experienced a fitness boom, this may now be reaching at least a temporary plateau in terms of the number of participants. On the other hand, those who do participate are seemingly becoming active more frequently. In Ontario, those exercising three or more times per week increased from 26% of the adult population in November 1978 to 32% in June 1979, 45% in June 1981, 37% in November 1981, 44% in June 1983, and 30% in November 1983 (Ontario Ministry of Tourism and Recreation, 1983; Tables 3.2 and 3.3). Moreover, no evidence exists to show that urban migration is inhibiting participation. Indeed, the proportion of active individuals is slightly lower

Table 3.2 Participation in Physical Activity

Frequency of Activity	November 1978 %	June 1979 %	November 1979 %	June 1983 %	November 1983 %
Three times per week	26	32	29	44	30
Once per week	23	20	21	18	23
Once per month	7	6	5	5	5
Inactive	44	42	44	32	43

Note. Based on data of Fitness Ontario, 1981, and unpublished data of Fitness Ontario, Ministry of Culture and Recreation, 1983.

Table 3.3 Time of Initiation of Exercise

Time of Initiation	November 1978 %	June 1979 %	November 1979 %	June 1983 %	November 1983 %
Last 6 months	14	20	10	14	15
Last 7-12 months	5	6	5	3	5
More than 1 year ago	81	74	85	83	80

Note. Based on data of Fitness Ontario, 1981, and unpublished data of Fitness Ontario, Ministry of Culture and Recreation, 1983.

in rural areas than in large cities (possibly because of a lower socio-economic status) (Table 3.4).

Currently the most popular activities (Statistics Canada, 1975, 1979b; Fitness Ontario, 1981; President's Council on Physical Fitness and Sports, 1973, May) are walking, calisthenics, jogging, swimming, and cycling, although in Canada skating and hockey tend to replace cycling during the winter months. Walking is particularly popular with women and with elderly subjects, while young men enjoy a wide range of activities. Data for individual activities show similar preferences and support the view that although interest increased in the early 1970s, a plateau of participation is now being approached. Between 1976 and 1981, the main Canadian growth was in cross-country skiing, alpine skiing, golf, and tennis, with respective increases of 142%, 69%, 32%, and 23% in the number of individuals reporting these activities at least once per year (Fitness & Amateur Sport, 1983b).

Some of the apparent plateau represents a broadened range of interests. Nevertheless, one might infer that the impact of government-sponsored promotional campaigns such as the President's Council on Physical Fitness, ParticipACTION, and Fitness Ontario has reached its peak and that in the absence of new promotional initiatives, penetration of the leisure market is virtually complete. Major arguments against such a viewpoint are the steep socioeconomic and age-related gradients of participation. Taking the Ontario data for November 1979 (activity at least once per month) and assuming that the enthusiasm of the blue-collar segment of the population could be brought to that of a university graduate (71% participation), the overall adult participation rate (currently 56%) would rise by 15%. A further 14% gain would occur if those over the age of 30 years became as active as those aged 18-29 years (70% participation rate averaged across social strata). Thus with appropriately directed advertising, a final participation rate of 88-89% might be achieved. This

Table 3.4 Influence of Education Upon Sport Participation by Adults*

Years of Schooling	Swimming %	Skating %	Tennis %	Golf %	Ice Hockey %	Cross-Country Skiing %	Downhill Skiing %	Curling %	Walking %	Gymnastics %
≤ 8	13	13	3	3	4	3	1	2	28	9
10	35	19	14	12	10	7	7	5	42	22
14	46	23	15	18	13	11	13	6	49	26
16	51	24	25	22	10	18	14	10	51	27
All categories	32	17	13	11	8	8	7	5	40	19

*Activities pursued at least once in past year.

Note. From "Schooling and Leisure Activities" by Y. Ferland, 1980, November (for a survey of 70,000 Canadians > 14 years conducted in 1976), *Canadian Statistical Review*, vi-ix.

would represent a tripling of present involvement, but nevertheless it seems to be an attainable objective.

Continued growth in the demand for active recreation over the next decade will undoubtedly be influenced heavily by changes in the pattern of employment (chapter 4). Current social trends suggest that not only an increase of unemployment may occur, but also that society may polarize into those with demanding work schedules and those with little or no regular work. Different tactics will thus be needed to reach these two distinct populations, and ultimately work-based fitness programs of the type reviewed in chapter 4 may bypass a large segment of society. It will also be necessary to make a clearer distinction between obligatory nonwork duties (which may be substantial among those with limited incomes due to unemployment), free time due to lack of employment, and leisure time (where resources are allocated, permitting the individual to pursue a voluntary activity of his or her choice). The likelihood that free time can be applied to the development of personal fitness may depend heavily upon its distribution—particularly whether the potential leisure period is available on a daily or a weekly basis or is concentrated at specific seasons of the year.

Purchase of Goods and Services

Recreation is claiming an increasing proportion of total personal budgets (Métivier, 1975; Willie, 1976, December; Walz, 1978; U.S. Dept. of Commerce, 1979; Wagner & Washington, 1982; Ellis, 1982). In Ontario the total volume of economic activity associated with sport, recreation, and fitness has been estimated at 9% of the gross domestic product (Ellis, 1982), equivalent to 200,000 person-years of direct and indirect employment.

Data on the purchase of recreational goods and services is unfortunately complicated by the inclusion of items that require little or no physical activity (e.g., the purchase of recreational vehicles or admission to spectator sports); Geiss, Hicks, and Londeree (1978) further argue that the option of buying what they termed "goods-intensive," labor-saving recreational equipment is a conscious selection of inferior health by the consumer. Nevertheless, the active component of recreation has become a multimillion dollar industry (Tables 3.5 and 3.6). Ellis (1982) took 42 specific sports and estimated the proportions of casual, moderate, and enthusiastic participants in Ontario and their corresponding annual expenditures; direct outlays totaled $1.24B for the 42 sports with a further expenditure of $100M on fitness, giving a total investment of $325 per worker-year. About 90% of the participants in fitness programs had only

Table 3.5 Distribution of Recreational and Leisure Expenditures (Average Individual Figures for All Families and Unattached Individuals, 1978)[a]

Expenditures	$	%
Outdoor recreation	462.4	30.5
Water sport	13.4	
Ski equipment	27.0	
Golf equipment	9.6	
Hockey (including skates)	19.5	
Tennis/badminton	5.9	
Other active sports	13.0	
Bicycles	31.5	
Camping and picnic equipment	14.7	
Vehicle purchase and operation	323.6	
Other passive recreation	4.2	
Admissions	121.8	8.0
Movies	51.4	
Plays and concerts	21.6	
Spectator sports	23.8	
Other	25.0	
Fees and licenses	102.4	6.8
Commercial	56.8	
Nonprofit	38.2	
Government	7.4	
Home recreation	254.4	16.8
Home entertainment	346.7	22.9
Reading	173.0	11.4
Other, including courses	55.3	3.6
	$1,516[b]	

[a]A few of the items show minor differences from the 1981 analysis of the same data.

[b]This total does not include purchases of recreational clothing. It is difficult to distinguish clothing fads from items actually related to physical activity, but a probable figure for sport clothing purchases is $106 per family.

Note. From *Family Expenditures in Canada* (pp. 178-179) by Statistics Canada, 1980, Occasional paper 62-550, Ottawa: Author.

Expressed in 1983 Canadian dollars.

a casual interest and spent an average of $9.38 per year; 8% of the moderate participants spent an average of $70 \cdot yr^{-1}$, and the remaining 2% of the enthusiasts spent $470 \cdot yr^{-1}$.

Much of the data concerning expenditures on recreational goods and services is expressed per family unit (Table 3.6). Unfortunately a combination of high divorce rates, family separations, and temporary unions is making the classical family with 1.9 children a somewhat dated con-

Table 3.6 Family Income, Disposable Income, and Consumer Prices for Recreation

Income and Prices	1961	1971	1973	1975	1977	1978	1979
Family income ($)	—	19,141	19,978	21,826	22,865	23,461	—
Disposable income ($)	5,507	7,784				10,484	10,674
Consumer prices[a] (1971 = 100)	75.0	100	112.7	138.5	160.8	175.1	191.2
Recreational prices[b] (1971 = 100)	—	100	107.1	128.5	142.7	148.2	158.4
Ratio of recreational to consumer prices	—	1.00	0.95	0.93	0.89	0.85	0.83
Ratio of disposable income to recreational prices (1971 = 100)	—	100	—	—	—	159	166

[a]From Table 1.3. Note that in terms of disposable income (1983 dollars) the C.P.I. = 100 throughout.

[b]For recreational items, reading, and education.

Note. From Travel, Tourism, and Outdoor Recreation—A Statistical Digest 1978 and 1979 (pp. 150-159), by Statistics Canada, 1981, Occasional paper 87-401, Ottawa: Statistics Canada.

cept. A need exists to develop statistics relating more specifically to single-parent families, single adults (living alone or as temporary couples), and elderly single or couple households. Ignoring these limitations, recreational expenditures in Canada currently amount to about $2300 per family; readily identified components due to active pursuits account for only about $324 per family-year, somewhat less than the Ellis (1982) figure. Costs are divided between equipment purchases (37.4%), athletic clothing (32.9%), admission fees to sporting facilities and events (26.7%), and the construction of private swimming pools (3.0%).

Measured in constant (1983) Canadian dollars, the average family more than doubled its expenditure on bicycles from 1969 to 1974, although part of this increase was attributable to a choice of more expensive models rather than the sale of more machines. The purchase of equipment for sports and games also increased by 74% over the same period. However, the total of recreational purchases has subsequently remained relatively static. This reflects, in part, a rapid growth and subsequent plateauing of disposable income (Table 3.6). During the period under review, the cost of many recreational goods and services declined as the volume of production increased and demand waned; by 1979 the ratio of disposable income to the cost of recreational products had improved 66%.

An analysis of 1974 data (MacLean-Hunter Research Bureau, 1977; Shephard, 1983b) indicates that only 8.1% of the typical family's $1212 recreational expenditure was spent on equipment for active pursuits (a total of $97.89, distributed between ski equipment, $33.38; boats, $19.26; golf, $12.77; and other equipment, $32.48). The 1978 figures (Table 3.6) show a similar picture. Out of a total recreational expenditure of $1516, $462.40 (30.5%) was spent on equipment for outdoor recreation and $119.90 (7.9%) was allocated to active pursuits. Unfortunately, this provides no guarantee that the equipment was used frequently or that the resultant intensity of activity was sufficient to improve fitness. In Norway, expenditures on active recreation ($167 per family-year) are of a similar order (Waaler & Hjort, 1982).

Clearly, scope is available in western countries for an increase in active recreational expenditures. Discretionary purchases that could well be curtailed include tobacco and alcoholic beverages (in Canada, currently nine times active recreation!), expensive recreational vehicles, and equipment for home entertainment. Total recreational expenditures climbed from $5.57B in 1971 to $9.29B in 1978 and remained a relatively static percentage of personal expenditures (Statistics Canada, 1981). Given a Canadian labor force of approximately 10 million, the total recreational expenditure would amount to $929 per worker (compare the estimate of $1516 per family, Table 3.6), $131 of which would be spent on sporting goods and accessories (rather higher than the estimate of $119.90 per family in Table 3.6, presumably because accessories were not included in the family total).

Details of fee receipts from Canadian recreational establishments (Table 3.7) suggest an expenditure of $786.6M per year, or, assuming 6.1 million family units, $129 per family, a figure of the same order as found in Table 3.6. Unfortunately, many of the items listed do not necessarily lead to enhanced physical activity. More than half of the total is attributable to membership in golf and country clubs, while other large items are admission fees for bowling alleys, ski facilities, and the rubric encompassing athletic clubs, arenas, stadiums, and athletic grounds. About 63.8% of fees accrue to commercial interests, 32.9% to nonprofit organizations, and 3.3% to various levels of government.

Data on the manufacture, import, export, and sale of recreational equipment are summarized in Table 3.8. In general, these figures confirm that interest in fitness and active recreation is currently at a plateau. The alternative hypothesis (that the community need for equipment has been satisfied) can be disproved (see Tables 3.9 and 3.10). Household ownership of most recreational equipment in recent years has increased only a little, and even wealthy households still lack most of the items needed for a varied recreational experience. Items where official figures suggest that the rate of manufacture has been maintained or is still increasing include cross-country ski packages, snowshoes, and sailboats. Even cross-country skiing may now have plateaued; a survey of visitors to 16 major courses in the Province of Quebec found that on average

Table 3.7 Receipts From Recreational Establishments

Type of Activity	1971 $	%
Golf and country clubs	457.2M	58.0
Athletic clubs, stadiums, arenas, and grounds	106.1M	13.5
Bowling alleys	94.4M	12.0
Ski facilities	62.2M	7.9
Curling clubs	28.0M	3.6
Riding academies	19.6M	2.5
Skating rinks	7.6M	1.0
Driving ranges and miniature golf courses	6.7M	0.9
Boat, canoe, and yacht rental	4.8M	0.6
Total	$786.6M	

Note. From *Travel, Tourism, and Outdoor Recreation 1973/74* (pp. 129-185) by Statistics Canada, 1975, Catalogue CS 66-202/1974, Ottawa: Statistics Canada.

Expressed in 1983 Canadian dollars.

Table 3.8 Manufacture, Import, and Sales Values of Specific Items of Recreational Equipment

Item	1966	1968	1970	1972	1974	1976	1977	1978
Bicycles (units)[a]	120K	239K	380K	1051K	723K	853K	784K	451K
($ value)	7.57M	13.88M	23.91M	89.15M	52.89M	56.56M	55.68M	34.61M
Ski packages (units)	34.5K	271K	346K	439K	686K	1083K	1296K	1337K
($ value)	7.57M	12.98M	20.18M	25.96M	32.56M	52.14M	51.96M	67.24M
Snowshoes (units)	—	—	—	—	115K	82K	—	109K
($ value)	0.90M	2.05M	1.45M	—	2.69M	2.55M	2.40M	2.68M
Golf clubs (sets)	—	—	—	—	1284K	843K	264K	449K
($ value)	—	—	—	26.39M	25.50M	18.68M	13.21M	11.57M
Hockey sticks (units)	—	—	—	8.20M	14.05M	5.10M	4.27M	3.71M
($ value)	12.38M	21.22M	26.48M	29.88M	35.98M	27.99M	26.57M	25.65M
Canoes (units)	9K	11K	17K	27K	33K	19K	12K	8K
($ value)	3.99M	4.44M	6.83M	10.67M	11.76M	7.45M	4.22M	2.83M
Rowboats (units)	8K	9K	9K	3K	17K	6K	4K	7K
($ value)	3.80M	4.92M	4.48M	1.49M	8.85M	3.03M	1.81M	4.58M
Sailboats (units)	—	—	—	5K	10K	6K	5K	6K
($ value)	—	—	—	46.49M	75.24M	55.34M	47.31M	63.63M
Snowmobiles (units)	79K	187K	363K	146K	123K	—	—	—
($ value)	—	—	—	292.9M	245.9M	—	—	—
Sum of all items ($) except snowmobiles	88.9M[b]	132.4M[b]	156.2M[b]	232.7M[c]	245.5M	223.7M	203.3M	212.8M

[a](Manufacture + import – export).

[b]Golf clubs and sailboats estimated at 1972 level.

[c]Snowshoes estimated at 1974 level.

Note. From *Culture Statistics—Recreational Activities* by Statistics Canada, 1976, Occasional paper 87-501, Ottawa: Statistics Canada and *Travel, Tourism, and Outdoor Recreation—A Statistical Digest 1978 and 1979* by Statistics Canada, 1981, Occasional paper 87-401, Ottawa: Author. Expressed in 1983 Canadian dollars. Note that calculations are based on shipments and ignore possible variations of inventory.

Table 3.9 Household Ownership of Selected Items of Recreational Equipment

Item	1971 %	1974 %	1976 %	1978 %
Skis	—	17.4	19.0	25.4
Canoe(s)	2.0	3.9	4.3	5.0
Rowboat(s)	2.9	2.8	3.4	˙3.4
Sailboat(s)	0.9	1.0	1.2	1.3
Adult bicycle(s)	(27.0)	41.6	39.1	41.9
Swimming pool	(3.8)	—	—	—
Snowmobile	—	9.3	9.8	9.7

Note. From *Travel, Tourism, and Outdoor Recreation—A Statistical Digest 1978 and 1979* (pp. 101-103) by Statistics Canada, 1981, Occasional paper 87-401, Ottawa: Statistics Canada; and MacLean Hunter Research Bureau, 1977.

Table 3.10 Influence of Family Income Upon Ownership of Selected Items of Recreational Equipment

Item	Income and Percent Ownership					All Subjects
	< 6K	6-12K	12-15K	15-25K	> 25K	
Skis						
Downhill	7	7	10	14	25	15
Cross-country	7	10	14	20	27	18
Canoe(s)	Z	3	4	6	9	6
Rowboat(s)	Z	3	3	4	6	4
Adult bicycle(s)	26	32	40	51	63	48
Snowmobile(s)	7	10	14	12	13	12

Note. From *Travel, Tourism, and Outdoor Recreation—A Statistical Digest 1978 and 1979* (pp. 101-103) by Statistics Canada, 1981, Occasional paper 87-401, Ottawa: Statistics Canada; and MacLean Hunter Research Bureau, 1977.

equipment had been purchased 5 or 6 years earlier (Chevalier, Garnier, & Girard, 1983).

For other pursuits, the decrease of sales has been more severe. By 1978, shipments of adult bicycles had dropped to 43% of the 1972 peak expenditure. Total purchases of equipment for all types of recreation were apparently down by about 13% in 1978 relative to the 1974 peak of $254.5M. A substantial proportion of many items of U.S. and Canadian recreational equipment such as skis and golf clubs is now imported. The multiplier effect for imported goods is relatively small, and in order to reap the full commercial benefit of any national fitness boom, the competitiveness of local companies must be increased or restrictions must be placed upon the import of recreational equipment.

The number of sporting goods stores in Canada approximately doubled from 1966 to 1971 (Statistics Canada, 1966, 1971). Some have become large chains (e.g., Frank Shorter now operates 2000 stores for the sale of running gear in the U.S.). An unacceptably large mark-up is noticeable on the retail sale of some fashionable items of recreational equipment. Thus the net shipments of skis to Canadian distributors had a wholesale worth of $32.56M in 1974, but retail sales for the same year amounted to $265.7M. Statistics for departmental stores are confounded by inclusion of luggage in the totals. Nevertheless, the trend apparently has been for an opening of specialty shops and departmental stores are capturing less than their share of the growing recreational market. The magnitude of some international sport manufacturing companies has become quite formidable. By 1980 Adidas produced 280,000 pairs of athletic shoes per day, employed 40,000 people in 40 countries, and had a total business volume of over 1 billion dollars (Bennett, Howell, & Simri, 1983). The growth of such multinational organizations has unfortunately forced many smaller but long-established national suppliers out of business.

Because the fitness boom is a recent phenomenon, attempting some calculation of the steady-state demand for equipment is interesting. Canadian bicycle imports totaled about 6.2 million units from 1966 to 1976. Allowing for 1.3 million two-bicycle households, 58% of these machines remained functional in 1976. Canoe shipments totaled 210,000 over the same period; 143,000 were shipped between 1971 and 1976, and household ownership increased by 128,000. This suggests that the average canoe has a greater longevity than a bicycle. In contrast, rowboat shipments (51,000 from 1971 to 1976) did little to increase household stocks. Two explanations of this finding are possible—either aluminum and fiberglass vessels have replaced decaying wooden crafts or most of the purchases are by fishing marinas. Current ownership of most types of recreational equipment still shows a marked socioeconomic gradient (Table 3.10). This seems to be more a matter of socially developed interests than of available funds because the gradient is least for one of the more expensive items (snowmobiles).

Employment Opportunities

One U.S. report (Henle, 1972) put the total number of full- and part-time recreational workers at 26 million. Much depends on the definition of a recreational worker, and in our present context Henle's figure is certainly a gross overestimate. Other U.S. writers noted 150,000 governmental and 500,000 private sector employees in 1968, with a further 40% increase to 1977 (Kraus, 1971; Jensen, 1977). In Canada the annual output of appropriately trained graduates from universities and community colleges is at least 4000; this matches reasonably well with the Statistics Canada estimate that recreational services provide direct employment to about 2.5% of Canadian workers, with a fairly rapid growth of the recreational labor force over the past decade (Table 3.11). Direct spin-off employment includes federal and state or provincial program administrators, those engaged in the manufacture and sale (Table 3.12) of sporting goods, those building both indoor and outdoor facilities (Table 3.13), and (less directly) those producing materials and supplies for equipment manufacturers (in which production accounts for approximately 47% of the wholesale cost of shipments).

Although active leisure is labor-intensive, much of the employment in recreational services is at a fairly modest salary. Nevertheless, assuming that many of the workers concerned would otherwise be unemployed, the difference between their average incomes and unemployment benefits provides a useful general stimulus to the economy. A further important consideration is that active leisure creates new job opportunities in certain regions traditionally affected by high rates of unemployment. This issue is considered further in the following section.

In the recent past, 7-14% of the capital cost of Canadian public recreational facilities has been met by the federal government; the residue has come from provincial, regional, and municipal coffers. Expenditures have amounted to 0.4-0.6% of the GNP. About three quarters of the total has been allocated to major spectator facilities (arenas, theatres, museums, and libraries), but investment has also increased in both park systems and outdoor recreational facilities such as swimming pools and tennis

Table 3.11 Employment in Recreational Services in Canada

Year	Employment Total	%
1974	224K	2.44
1975	232K	2.48
1976	243K	2.55
1977	250K	2.57
1978	261K	2.63

Note. Based on data of Canada Year Book, 1980-81.

Table 3.12 Possible Economic Consequences of Activity for All Adult Canadians, Expressed as Required Annual Totals of Additional Expenditure

Source of Expenditure	Amount ($)
Facilities	
Governmental investment	438M
Private sector investment	73M
(Direct construction work $188M per year; also access roads and utility services)	
Equipment and supplies	
Recreational equipment	1,757M
Recreational clothing	641M
Recreational admission fees	661-1,574M[a]
(Major benefit to distributors, retail trade, and real estate)	
Operation and maintenance	
500,000 additional workers	3,000M
(Costs partly offset by decrease of unemployment and taxes paid)	
Other	
Potential increase of food consumption (see ch. 2)	503M

[a]Values with and without membership in golf and country clubs (58% of recreational admissions).

Expressed in 1983 Canadian dollars.

Table 3.13 Construction Work Generated by Building Outdoor Recreational Facilities

Year	Amount	Year	Amount
1971	28.6M	1976	54.4M
1972	38.5M	1977	68.3M
1973	32.0M	1978	91.8M
1974	111.8M	1979	90.5M
1975	58.4M	1980	94.2M

Note. From *Travel, Tourism and Outdoor Recreation—A Statistical Digest 1978 and 1979* (p. 181) by Statistics Canada, 1983, Occasional paper 87-401, Ottawa: Statistics Canada.

Expressed in 1983 Canadian dollars.

courts. With the possible exceptions of golf and downhill skiing, participants rely heavily upon the availability of publicly owned facilities, and this factor merits careful consideration when assessing future needs for the public ownership of recreational land (Tables 3.14 and 3.15).

Table 3.14 Type of Facility Used for Various Sports

Type of Facility	Swimming %	Ice Skating %	Tennis %	Golf %	Type of Sport Ice Hockey %	Cross-Country Skiing %	Downhill Skiing %
Public recreational	34.2	68.5	54.7	35.1	68.3	26.3	42.6
At work or at school	3.3	2.1	8.9	1.8	3.3	3.4	—
Outside—no special facility	22.7	10.5	5.4	2.7	7.3	43.0	6.6
Commercial/club	8.5	4.2	14.4	49.8	7.3	3.1	—
At home	11.7	2.0	2.9	—	1.8	8.2	38.1

Note. From *Culture Statistics—Recreational Activities* (p. 48) by Statistics Canada, 1976, Occasional paper 87-501, Ottawa: Statistics Canada.

Table 3.15 Relative Contribution of Public and Private Sectors to Various Leisure Facilities in the Area Administered by the British Greater London Council

Facility	Public %	Private %
Ten-pin bowling	0	100
Ice skating rinks	0	100
Squash centers	10	90
Sports centers	71	29
Indoor swimming baths	100	0
Outdoor swimming baths	96	4
Tennis courts	46	54
Golf courses	28	72
Football pitches	70	30
Athletic tracks	83	17
Cycle tracks	100	0

Note. Based on data of Greater London Recreation Study, 1976.

Activity For All

At present, about a quarter of North American adults claim to be exercising adequately (three or more times per week), a quarter participate in some activity, and a half are inactive (Table 3.1). The data also show a strong age gradient. Thus the Canada Health Survey (1982) found that 46% of men and 34% of women aged 15-19 years were very active, but in those aged 65 years and over the corresponding figures were only 11% of men and 5% of women.

If almost all of the population (perhaps 87%) could be motivated to an appropriate level of physical activity, at least a threefold increase of recreational expenditures might be anticipated. The problem is not knowing how far such expenditures could be realized in practice, because physical activity is not necessarily proportional to expense, and the majority of those who are currently inactive lack a large margin of disposable income. Both tastes and the financial ability to accommodate such tastes become less certain as recreational activity is extended to include the lower socioeconomic strata. Moreover, current popular pursuits of the average North American (walking, jogging, swimming, cycling, and gardening) all provide less stimulus to the economy than more exotic sports. Nevertheless, a recent study from Sault Sainte Marie showed that a high local unemployment rate (> 30%) had increased rather than diminished the demand for recreational facilities. Despite a severe shortage of cash, the local population apparently continued to invest in active leisure.

Facilities

Provision of extra facilities may be hampered by high land costs (Shephard, 1977b). Much of the existing recreational land in North America and western Europe was acquired many years ago. If participation showed a sudden threefold jump, many facilities would become unpleasantly crowded. On the more likely assumption of a slow move toward target participation, needs could possibly be satisfied by tripling the current rate of investment in parks and recreational facilities. Making this simple assumption, an expense of $40-50 per worker-year would need to be met by some combination of admission fees, increases in personal taxation, reduced health-care costs, and diversion of funds from massive spectator projects.

If commercial resources continue to satisfy about one seventh of facility needs, an annual $73M of additional investment would also be required per year in the construction of privately operated recreational facilities.

One of the prime beneficiaries of such a new investment would be the construction industry. During the fiscal year 1981-82, Australia saw the equivalent of about $31M invested in constructing and equipping new health and fitness centers (Wilson, 1981, November 8-14). In Canada a tripling of investment would generate direct construction of $188M per year, although the building of access roads and installing of utility services (electricity, gas, water, sewers) could augment this figure substantially.

The British Sports Council views central government investment in facilities as a form of seed money. For example, an expenditure of $56 million on sport centers is expected to stimulate an investment of $86 million by voluntary bodies and $298 million by local municipalities (an immediate four- to fivefold "gearing" effect). Canadian statistics suggest an even larger gearing of governmental investment. Squash courts are a controversial component of public spending, but in the British example such facilities are justified as a means of generating operating income for sport centers (Scottish Sports Council, 1980).

Equipment

A threefold increment of equipment purchases would see each Canadian family spending an additional $240 per year on recreational equipment. About $88 worth of recreational clothing and up to $215 worth of admission to recreational establishments would be added to this. The total of $543 per family amounts to about 5% of disposable income. If found by a uniform reduction in the purchase of other nonessential items, it would have a barely noticeable effect upon other sectors of the market place, particularly if the resultant reduction of unemployment led to a general stimulation of economic activity.

When people are faced with a shrinking disposable income, the recreational sector is commonly curtailed. A survey by the U.S. magazine, *Changing Times* (1974), found that 59% of a 25,000-person sample had reduced recreational spending to counter inflation; other targets were eating out (52%), purchasing major appliances (48%), and paying rent (3%). Likewise, much of any increase in expenditures on active leisure would draw upon disposable income.

A specific increase of active recreational expenditures could have a very beneficial indirect influence upon health if it was accommodated by a corresponding reduction in the sale of tobacco and alcohol. Some multinational corporations have protected themselves against this contingency by hedging investments in tobacco and breweries with parallel investments in leisure industries. Other likely targets for reduced consumption in a more active population are recognized in some corporate structures (Roberts, 1979); items that have been identified include admissions to movies, purchases of sedentary recreational equipment such as snowmobiles, indoor hobbies and entertainment (including television advertising), reading material, and dress clothing.

It would be useful to examine specifically the impact of enhanced physical activity upon spectator sport. In the U.S., ticket sales and concessions currently gross over $2 billion per year. The construction of stadia has played a major role in many recent municipal, state or provincial, and federal budgets. The capital cost of the New Orleans Superdome (1975) amounted to the current equivalent of $386 million, while the fiberglass-roofed Silverdome in Pontiac, MI, cost the equivalent of $94 million. Although commonly promoted as an investment in regional economies, 83% of publicly owned stadia in the U.S. show an operating loss. In 20% of the installations, this amounts to more than $2.3 M • yr^{-1}, and subsidization of teams are particularly large in the biggest stadia (Noll, 1974).

Bennett et al. (1983) put the cost of the Munich Olympic Games ($600 million) at $30,000 per minute, and in Montreal costs were even higher (Bellefleur, 1976).

Despite these heavy subsidies, the relative financial health of commercial sport is indicated by the current value of various teams and the annual salaries of individual players. Over the first 6 years of its operation, a San Diego football team (the Chargers) grossed the current equivalent of $48M in ticket sales, $33M in national television revenues, and $16.7M in receipts from away games and had additional income from food concessions (net $0.77M), parking (net $0.90M), and local television and radio companies (Love, 1973, October/November). In cities where a substantial demand exists for admission, the profits from professional teams can equal 25-50% of gross revenues (McPherson, 1975). Both the costs and profits from spectator sports are typically lower in Canada, partly because existing stadia are smaller than in the U.S. Nevertheless, the usual magnitude of takings is such that government must look very critically at requests to subsidize the capital and operating costs of spectator sports, irrespective of whether the demand for such leisure pursuits increases or decreases (Kowet, 1977).

Who would be the major beneficiaries of a renewed boom in active recreational expenditures? Given the six-to eightfold markup on most types of equipment, a large part of anticipated equipment sales (about $200 per worker-year) would accrue to the distributive and retail trades. However, manufacturers of sport equipment and clothing and real estate operators would also benefit from the opening of new sport goods and cycle stores.

Major recipients of admission fees in North America (Table 3.7) are golf and country clubs. It is by no means certain that people who are presently inactive would consider membership in such an establishment as essential to their developments of personal exercise programs. If the golf and country club item is eliminated, extra admission fees for an active society would drop to $90 per family, a total of $661M.

Employment

Vickerman (1975) estimated that in North Wales the job-creating potential of unit recreational investment was 2.29 times the typical figure for the United Kingdom (U.K.) (cost per job $8601, compared with the average of $19,691). Ellis (1982) put the immediate cost of an average Canadian recreational worker at $22,300 (wage, salary, and benefit costs). He further suggested a need for two part-time positions per full-time recreational worker and an employment multiplier effect of 2.17 for the recreational appointments.

The current distribution of the Canadian labor force is summarized in Table 3.16. Given a tripling of popular interest in physical activity and the demand for recreational services and administration, together with the manufacture, distribution, and sale of recreational equipment and clothing, employment would probably be generated for an extra 500,000-600,000 Canadians (5-6% of the labor force). Employment in planning, design, and construction should be added to this total, including immediate facilities (about 5000 workers), retail stores selling recreational goods, factories manufacturing recreational equipment, recreational resi-

Table 3.16 Approximate Distribution of Canadian Labor Force

Type of Work	1951 Number	1951 %	1971 Number	1971 %	1981† Number	1981† %
White-collar	1.67M	31.6	3.56M	41.3	4.36M	41.8
Managerial		8.0		7.9		6.1ᵃ
Professional and technical		7.3		12.5		14.8ᵇ
Clerical		11.0		14.8		15.8ᶜ
Sales		5.4		6.1		5.1ᵈ
Blue-collar	1.66M	31.4	2.20M	25.6	2.40M	22.9
Craft and production workers		24.7		20.8		18.4ᵉ
Laborers		6.6		4.7		4.5ᶠ
Transport and communications	0.33M	6.3	0.43M	5.0	0.85M	8.1
Service and recreation*	0.51M	9.7	1.00M	11.6	1.38M	13.2ᵍ
Primary occupations	1.05M	19.8	0.64M	7.5	0.75M	7.2
Farming		15.6		5.8		4.8
Logging		1.9		0.6		0.7
Fishing and trapping		1.0		0.3		0.7
Mining and quarrying		1.2		0.7		1.7ʰ
Other	0.06M	1.2	0.78M	9.0	0.72M	6.9ʲ
Total	5.28M		8.61M		10.46M	

†Some of the Bank of Canada categories apparently differ somewhat from Statistics Canada, as noted:

ᵃPublic administration and defense ᶠConstruction
ᵇNoncommercial services ᵍCommercial services
ᶜTrade ʰIncludes milling
ᵈFinance, insurance, and real estate ʲUnpaid work
ᵉManufacturing

*Only about a sixth of this total are employed in recreational services.

Note. Based on data of Canada Year Book, 1980-81, excluding Yukon and North West Territories.

dences, access roads, and utility installations. Spinoff employment could also be envisaged in service industries (restaurants, hotels, and gas stations), while other sectors of the economy might be stimulated less directly by the rise of purchasing power among the groups already named.

An input/output analysis for a British recreational system (Vickerman, 1975) suggested that the multiplier effect of recreational expenditures was fairly small (1.11, versus the national average of 2.58). Likewise, for the Province of Ontario (Berger, 1983), multiplier effects were set at 1.12 for athletic clothing, 1.16 for active recreational expenditures, 1.54 for provincial government expenditures (e.g., on provincial parks), and 1.88 for travel/accommodation. Multipliers for clothing and equipment were relatively low because much of the material purchased had been manufactured outside of the province. A second calculation suggested that every dollar the province invested in recreation stimulated $4.60 of direct private expenditures on active recreation, athletic clothing, vacations, and travel, with a further yield of $4.00 through the composite provincial multiplier and $0.47 through the donation of volunteer time (a total return of $9.07). Moreover, about 9.5 cents of every recreational dollar spent by the province was recouped as taxation (Ellis, 1982).

In some sports, the yield per dollar has been greater. Thus a provincial investment of $316,000 in speed-skating and ringette was associated with total direct expenditures of $4.1M. By way of comparison, the total return upon provincial investment in cultural facilities and the performing arts has been estimated at $2.60-3.60 per dollar, while specific investment in provincial parks has yielded a total return of less than $3.00 per dollar (Berger, 1983). Governmental support of local agencies delivering sport and fitness programs is important not only for the budgets of such organizations, but also as a means of fostering local agencies' acceptance in the community.

The economic impact of enhanced physical activity is particularly large in rural, recreation-based economies. A study of the northeastern part of the U.S. (U.S. Bureau of Outdoor Recreation, 1972) estimated that each recreational homeowner spent the current equivalent of $7480 per year in the tourist region; the total impact upon the regional economy was put at 1.55 times this figure (that is, $11,600 per homeowner-year). Such expenditures have important implications for disadvantaged indigenous populations in many countries.

While most "developed" nations would regard a 5-6% increase of employment as a most attractive prospect at the present juncture, economists will be quick to point out that, with the possible exception of alterations in the external balance of payments, recreational work does not create new capital. In the Canadian example, all of the likely additional 500,000 employees are concentrated in a service industry. At a salary of $14,500 per worker, the minimum cost to society would be a total of $8.34B in wages and fringe benefits. This might well be transferred from some other sector of the economy, although it could also be generated by increased production in automated factories. At least half of the required $8.34B would be met by a reduction of unemployment and welfare rolls, while a further 10-15% would immediately be returned to the government in taxation. Other contributions to the balance sheet might come from such areas as reductions in health-care costs (chapter 2). At most, the new expense (< $3B) would require a 1% rise of national productivity. Because a reduction of absenteeism and an increase of productivity are likely consequences of enhanced physical activity (chapter 4), the required 1% gain of output seems to be a realistic assumption, even if there is not a major investment in robotics.

Details of costs per unit of employment can be illustrated by the experience of a regional conservation authority near Toronto (Table 6.6). An annual expenditure of $541,800 on the park facility currently generates the direct equivalent of 7 + (6 × 15/52), or 8.7 full-time positions—a cost of about $62,000 per worker. However, the employment potential of the park is substantially larger than 8.7 positions and has scope for additional swimming, skiing, life-saving, and natural history instructors. Moreover, such staff could be added for about $18,850 per individual (salary and fringe benefits), marginally less than the $20,000 per worker-year currently quoted for make-work projects. At the same time, the benefits to the employee (continuing work) and to the community (greater recreational activity) would justify a recreational approach to unemployment in terms of its health and social value, even if administrative costs were to push the total expense above the make-work figure of $20,000 per employee-year.

Whether full participation of the population in physical activity would yield the postulated 5-6% increase of employment depends in part upon the impact of other benefits of exercise upon the labor market. If medical care costs are reduced, for example, there may be some countereffect from a reduction of the labor force employed in hospitals and nursing homes. However, given the age profile of most western nations, the consequence of improved personal health most likely will be a containment rather than a curtailment of medical and hospital sector employment.

Balance Sheet

A balance sheet for a more active society (Table 3.12) suggests that the capital investment in new facilities could be offset by additional recreational admission fees. This would leave the recreational consumer to meet the costs of recreational equipment, clothing, admissions, and food (about 5% of disposable income); the government would cover the new costs of the additional workers involved in operation and maintenance of recreational facilities (about 1% of GNP).

Capacity Versus Demand in Physical Activity Facilities

An earlier review (Shephard, 1977b) noted that active people were able to enjoy their present patterns of exercise because of the inactivity of their fellow citizens. This chapter will be concluded by examining the impact of a threefold increase of current activity patterns upon the demand for physical facilities.

Plainly, in many countries municipal recreational facilities are operating at capacity during peak hours. Swimming pools are overcrowded to the point that users must wait for admission, skating arenas are open into the small hours of the morning, some of the larger urban parks have grass worn thin from overuse, and supposed wilderness areas are deteriorating from a combination of carelessness and excessive occupancy. The only remedy is thus to increase the number of recreational facilities, realizing much of the anticipated new construction discussed above.

Some countries lack the necessary land to expand recreational opportunities. Lakefront and wilderness areas within easy driving distance of large cities are in especially short supply. If wilderness experience was accepted as an important part of the total recreational package, it would probably be necessary to establish residential camps in remote areas so that city-dwellers could visit such locations for 1- or 2-week vacations.

Urban areas have substantial tracts of land that could be used for the construction of swimming pools, skating arenas, and even small parks. Possibilities include disused railway sidings and factories, urban redevelopment areas, gravel pits, sanitary landfill sites, and lakeshore reclamation. Finance is one major obstacle to such acquisitions.The high cost of urban land is, in part, real—a response to world population pressures—but it is also, in part, artificial—a consequence of extensive purchases by a small group of entrepreneurial developers. The cost of recreational facilities (chapter 6) could thus be substantially reduced by legislation that firmly restricted speculation in land holdings.

The impact of increased recreational development upon tourism is likely to be positive. While a small proportion of travelers are seeking unspoiled wilderness, the majority wish to enjoy an active vacation. A study in Ontario (Berger, 1983) noted that participation in sporting events or outdoor activities occurred in 24% of all trips over 40 km in length, while recreation and/or pleasure were primary motivations in 35% of all trips. If there were more ''things to do,'' a holiday would thus become correspondingly more attractive.

Conclusions

Cost-effectiveness and cost-benefit calculations must be tempered by a variety of sociocultural considerations. Government must decide how far activity habits are molded by the social climate rather than by personal decisions. The effectiveness of exercise needs to be weighed critically against other potential lifestyle expenditures, particularly measures to check smoking. Such analysis should take particular account of likely response rates—not only among those currently interested in exercise, but also among inactive target groups.

Available data suggest that while physical activity has become more prevalent over the past decade, in many sports and pastimes at least a temporary plateau of participation has now been reached. Scope is available for repeating and expanding the surveys that currently document public exercise behavior, taking care that questionnaire responses remain compatible with previous investigations. The price markup on recreational equipment merits careful scrutiny, and the psychosocial impact of over-priced sporting goods upon the exercise habits of both rich and poor people needs to be evaluated. The potential to triple employment in the recreational sector through the promotion of physical activity for all deserves particularly careful attention. If recreational expenditures are increased, which areas of discretionary expenditure will be curtailed? In particular, will demands for spectator sport increase or decrease? Will the promise of new jobs be realized, or will much of the potential benefit be dissipated by a curtailing of activity in other sectors of the market place? Answers to each of these questions seem likely to emerge over the next 10 years.

chapter 4

Industrial Consequences
of Enhanced Physical Fitness

It is in the interests of employers as well as of the community to maintain a fit and effective work force . . . (employers should) consider the provision of sport and recreational facilities for use by their employees at breaks or after work. (Department of Health and Social Security, 1977)

The impact of automation, wildly fluctuating oil prices, and displacement of industry to emerging third-world countries makes it quite hazardous to predict either the future performance of the economy or how it might be enhanced by personal fitness. However, a substantial amount of data that assesses the influence of physical activity upon such current statistics as worker satisfaction, productivity, absenteeism, turnover, and industrial injuries is available. Tangible benefits to both employers and employees have been inferred (Bjurstrom & Alexiou, 1978; Martin, 1978; Wilbur, 1983), although some authors have been critical of these claims (Haskell & Blair, 1980; Fielding, 1982; Pate & Blair, 1983).

Physical Activity and Automation

One possible model for a national economy is illustrated in Figure 4.1. It seems almost inevitable that the next 2 decades will witness a progressive decline of conventional manufacturing in most western nations. This will reflect, in part, a displacement of work to third-world countries, and, in part, the influence of automation.

The rate of extraterritorial displacement of industry depends on several factors, including (a) the fiscal advantage of relocation, as seen by multinational corporations (e.g., differentials in wage rates, union regulations, safety and health requirements, tax incentives), and (b) governmental investment incentives (e.g., trade agreements, tariff barriers, tax concessions). Given the number of variables involved, estimating the rate

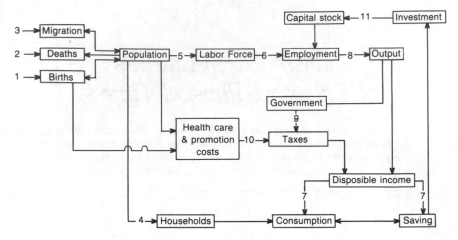

Figure 4.1 A possible basis for modeling changes in the Canadian economy with particular reference to health care and promotion. The balance of the model is influenced by (1) fertility rates, (2) death rates, (3) migration rates, (4) number of independent households, (5) participation in the labor force, (6) unemployment, (7) consumption versus saving, (8) productivity, (9) government policies and expenditures, (10) health care costs, and (11) depreciation of capital stock. Improved health could influence (1), (2), (3), (4), (5), (7), (8), and (10), while increased physical activity might also modify (6), (9), and (11). *Note.* Based on concepts from ''Health Care Costs When the Population Changes'' by F. Denton and B. Spencer, 1980b, In V.W. Marshall (Ed.), *Aging in Canada. Social Perspectives* (pp. 232-247), Toronto: Fitzhenry and Whiteside.

of de-industrialization of a specific region is difficult; nevertheless, it must be assumed that the present trends will continue and indeed are likely to accelerate.

The rate of automation depends, in part, on governmental policies (tax incentives for increases of productivity vs. tariff barriers that conserve or fossilize existing levels of technology). The process is further influenced by the surplus of capital available for investment (this is dependent on the general buoyancy of the economy, the extent to which tax regulations favor investment, and the age profile of the population, chapter 1). Again, estimating the rate of change is dangerous, but it can be assumed that the current trend toward automation will continue and even accelerate, whether production is publicly or privately owned. Professor Henry Levine of Stanford University (unpublished) has predicted that robots and computer software will displace 3 million U.S. workers over the next 20 years and a continuation of the trend will lead to a loss of 8 million positions by the year 2025. This amounts to an 8% direct growth of unemployment with the likelihood that an associated "ripple" will cause a total loss of 10-14% of existing jobs.

Another imponderable concept is how long the economy can generate new jobs to make good losses from displacement and automation. The margin of unemployment is also influenced by the growth of the labor force. For the next few years the number of North Americans seeking work will increase due to of a combination of (a) a decrease in the proportion of full-time homemakers, (b) a decrease in the proportion of school-age dependents, and (c) a continuing migration of people from less-developed countries. However, toward the end of the present century, the size of the North American labor force will stabilize or even decline unless major changes take place in immigration or retirement policies. The ability to create new jobs depends partly upon the supply of capital (discussed earlier) and partly upon the manner in which capital is invested. For example, if priority is assigned to the exploration of off-shore and Arctic oil fields, such activity will demand large amounts of capital but generate relatively little employment.

Investment in leisure programing has at least three attractions to those concerned about employment opportunities:

1. In common with other service industries, leisure programing is labor-intensive and thus will contribute directly to the growth of needed employment opportunities over the next 2 decades (chapter 3).
2. Leisure programing is likely to have a positive effect upon health (chapter 2) and therefore industrial performance (this chapter).
3. Leisure programing makes meaningful provision for those who, by choice or force of circumstances, have increased free time.

The last objective is plainly important to the health of modern society, although any cost-benefit evaluation of this item is likely to be a personal judgment.

Investment in leisure may be made through community recreational programs, employee fitness programs in government-controlled offices or factories, and employee fitness programs in private enterprises. Many corporations are becoming convinced of the value of on-site fitness (Pyle, 1979; Rodale, 1983; Wear, 1983). One fairly recent survey of the top 500 companies in the U.S. showed that 50% of the companies had established fitness programs over the previous 4 years, while a third planned to build or extend facilities over the next 2 years (Bennett et al., 1983, p. 161). Another recent writer (Andresky, 1982, December) estimated that 500 major U.S. firms provided some type of health facility, ranging from simple shower and exercise rooms to the 3440 m², $3.2M complex of the Kimberley Clark Corporation with its pool, sauna, and suspended 100 m track. In Japan, the Ministry responsible for fitness programing claims that 63.5% of companies with more than 30 workers currently have sport clubs for their employees (Ministry of Education, Science & Culture, 1981), while Sweden has 14,000 company athletic clubs (Bennett et al., 1983).

Despite pleas of altruism on the part of many entrepreneurs who make such investments, the industrial economics now to be discussed are also of interest to companies as they develop employee fitness policies.

Worker Satisfaction

The satisfaction of the average citizen is a complex issue (Watson, 1980; Shephard, 1984) and thus will not be reviewed in detail here. In some police states such as Poland and South Africa, the association between personal dissatisfaction and poor industrial performance is obvious to even a casual visitor. The potential sources of dissatisfaction for the U.S. (and to a lesser extent the Canadian) worker have been detailed in "Work in America" (1973). While the conclusions reached in this document have been strongly criticized (Shephard, 1984), the question remains as to whether an increase of worker satisfaction could improve industrial performance.

One survey (Wanzel, 1974) showed that 69% of Canadian workers believe that the introduction of a company-based employee fitness/lifestyle program would boost morale. Likewise, in the U.S. Groves (1980) suggested that an employee recreational program provided an integrating device and allowed a frank exchange of ideas between various strata of employees, which led to the development of common goals in a cooperative atmosphere.

Certainly, many corporations have made substantial improvements in the conditions of employment over the past decade. Innovations often include the provision of exercise facilities, but because of the complexity of the total package of policy alterations, the extent that an increase in physical activity has contributed to the resultant gains of industrial performance is uncertain.

Measures that are currently being adopted include "quality of working life" programs, relaxation breaks, fitness and lifestyle programs, and employee assistance programs with a strong emphasis upon personal counseling; the last type of activity falls outside the scope of this book.

Quality of Working Life Programs

The Swedish shipyard Kochum Mekaniska Verstadt A.B. provides one widely cited example where the overall working environment has been upgraded. The company, which has about 5,800 employees, decided in 1970 to replace a part-time industrial physician with a full-time occupational health unit employing two doctors, a dentist, and a physiotherapist. Workers were also allowed much greater autonomy on the shop floor. Interpersonal relations were fostered through the construction of well-styled dining rooms, lounges, saunas, and showers for groups of 40-100 workers, while a $5 million recreation complex was built for employees and their families. The immediate financial results of the company were good. The annual balance sheet shifted progressively from a loss of $13 million in 1970 to a 15% profit in 1973. Labor turnover (previously 50% per annum) also showed a dramatic decrease (Banister, 1978). However, attribution of the benefit is uncertain because no control company was evaluated over the same period.

Rosow (1977) described the effects of introducing a similar work enrichment program into an Indiana company that manufactured prefabricated buildings. Turnover dropped from 35 to 10-12% per year, and absenteeism dropped from the U.S. national average (4-5%) to 1.2%.

Relaxation Breaks

Some observers have argued that the benefits of an exercise class stem largely from a change in the pattern of activity rather than an increase of energy expenditure. Thus comments about a "relaxation break" are interesting.

Peters, Benson, and Porter (1977) examined 56 nonparticipants and 126 volunteers in a large manufacturing company. After 4 weeks of observation, volunteers were assigned randomly to one of three groups— (a) those given no instructions, (b) those allowed to attend relaxation classes, and (c) those taught specific relaxation techniques. Over the next 12 weeks, scores were kept for symptoms (30 somatic and 20 behavioral items), illnesses (pain or fever), work performance (4 items), sociability and satisfaction (6 items), and happiness. All measurements except the index of happiness improved roughly in proportion to involvement in the relaxation program.

Some authors have made quite strong financial claims for stress reduction methodology. Thus Manuso (1983) estimated that a biofeedback-centered relaxation program could save as much as 80% of the company costs arising from industrial stress, with a $5.52 return on every dollar invested.

It may be concluded that both quality of work life and relaxation programs have some practical value in the workplace and deserve consideration as alternatives, or preferably as adjuncts, to physical activity enhancement programs.

Fitness and Lifestyle Programs

Commonly, fitness and lifestyle programs have been introduced in a semialtruistic fashion through the personal enthusiasm of a physically active corporation president. Gains of physical and mental health, reduction of turnover and absenteeism, improved job efficiency, and better morale have often been anticipated, but, at least until recently, formal evaluation of fiscal benefits has not been attempted (Heinzelmann, 1975). Analysts have been intimidated by uncertainties regarding the time frame over which production and health benefits should be sought. Moreover, it has been argued that sophisticated discounting techniques are needed to adjust for likely changes in the value of future benefits and costs (Klarman, 1974; Sugden, 1978; Drummond, 1980). It has further been unclear how possible benefits should be apportioned between the company, taxpayers, and workers. Finally, the altruists have stressed that corporate health and fitness programs are not really set up to make profits (Jacobs & Chovil, 1983). On occasion exercise facilities are indeed conceived as a means of providing untaxed financial benefits to senior management (Alchian & Kessel, 1977; Atherley et al., 1976), and in such circumstances the impact on either company profits or the national economy becomes extremely hard to measure.

Nevertheless, in the long run any company must be assured that its programs are cost-effective, and its enthusiasm for a health promotion program will be enhanced if it can be shown at least to be breaking even. Recent cost scrutiny has suggested that an annual health examination for senior executives is not cost-effective (Wright, 1982). Likewise, single intervention programs that treat such problems as hypertension or obesity are at best only marginally cost-effective. The optimum tactic is to combine an enhancement of physical activity with a multiphasic attack on other health problems, thereby reducing high overhead costs (Collings, 1982).

Evaluation of the benefits of exercise is further complicated by the fact that positive findings are more likely to have been reported than negative data. Heinzelmann (1975) made a controlled comparison of exercisers and control subjects; 60% of those assigned to the physical activity group reported positive changes in work performance, compared with 3% of the control group. Specific comments included an ability to work harder (both physically and mentally) and improved powers of concentration and decision-making. About 40% of the active group developed more positive feelings toward their work, including a sense of greater energy and productivity and a lessening of boredom. Perceived health also improved, with a decrease of strain and tension, a lessening of cigarette consumption, and an improved quality of rest and sleep. Similar benefits were noted among employees of the U.S. National Aeronautics and Space Administration (NASA) who had been recruited to an on-site fitness facility (Heinzelmann, 1975).

Wilbur (personal communication) described the progressive introduction of a comprehensive fitness/lifestyle process at various locations of the U.S. Johnson and Johnson Company. Before introduction of the scheme, sick-leave amounted to 9.3h • yr^{-1} in those with no lifestyle problems but jumped to 20.3h • yr^{-1} in those who were unfit. This implies a potential to save about \$36 • yr^{-1} through the introduction of an exercise program (assuming an annual salary of \$14,500, a replacement cost of 1.75 times base salary, and 20% participation in a fitness/lifestyle program). If the employee also smoked, the annual time loss increased to 21.9h • yr^{-1}. With excess body fat it increased to 24.6h • yr^{-1}, and with poor stress management it increased to 35.8h • yr^{-1}. Participation in the lifestyle process increased health knowledge by 9% at 1 year (compared with 4% in control subjects). Alcohol problems decreased by 18% (0% in controls), 16% of subjects stopped smoking (4% of controls), and the fitness/lifestyle process also had favorable effects upon weight control, stress management, and hypertension. Self-reports indicated enhanced interpersonal relations, greater organizational commitment, easier handling of job strain, greater self-esteem on the job, and greater satisfaction with opportunities for personal growth.

Other U.S. corporations have reported similar findings (Andresky, 1982). Boeing found "obvious improvements . . . in self-esteem and job attitudes," and Hospital Corporation of America found an improvement of self-image in 86% of program participants (with 76% of subjects also noting more productivity at home). Bonnie Bell commented that exercisers "felt more positive about themselves," and at Rolm, employees started "to understand they're responsible for their lives."

A pilot fitness project at a government office in Ottawa (Slee & Peepre, 1974, May) noted improved work performance in 59% of the women. The attitude toward work was improved in 58% of the sample, and 78% reported less strain and tension after enrollment in the program. However, no controls were included. Marteniuk (personal communication) commented on decreased anxiety and enhanced work performance after introducing a fitness/lifestyle project to a refrigerator manufacturing plant. Layman (1972) and Howard, Cunningham, and Rechnitzer (1975) also ascribed mental health benefits to exercise programs.

A 17-week program at the head office of Ontario Hydro (Knezevich, 1980) involved about 20% of the employees. Physiological results included a 26.4% gain of predicted maximum oxygen intake and a 2.6% decrease in body fat. Self-reports suggested an increase in job satisfaction in 76% of the employees, an improved self-image in 94% of the employees, relief of stress in 92% of the employees, and an improvement in self-confidence in 90% of the employees. Both general and specific measures of work satisfaction were applied in a Toronto study of Life Assurance workers (Cox et al., 1981). On the scale of Smith, Kendal, and Hulin (1969), male employees were initially satisfied with their employments except in the areas of pay and promotions. Anxiety levels (Taylor scale) were low, self-image was stable, and relatively few major life events had occurred (scale of Holmes & Rahe, 1967) in the preceding year. The main changes after introduction of the fitness/lifestyle program at one of two matched companies were (a) a high incidence of life events in program dropouts and (b) a decrease in work-related events in high adherents to the program. High adherents also developed a more positive attitude toward physical activity, particularly with regard to its impact upon health and fitness.

The possible extent of program benefit inevitably varies with initial dissatisfaction; production-line work such as car manufacturing is particularly dissatisfying. The Ford Motor plant in Oakville, Ontario, noted a dramatic drop in the number of cars returned for warranty repairs following institution of careful programing to enhance the quality of working life.

The satisfied worker is less likely to disrupt productivity and generate health-care costs through personal abuse of tobacco, alcohol, and other drugs. In the Toronto Life Assurance study, the program led to a decrease in tobacco and alcohol use. However, possibly because the group was initially quite satisfied with its employment, changes of job satisfaction among participants in the employee fitness/lifestyle program were relatively small.

Employee Assistance Programs

Some companies have noted very substantial gains from employee assistance programs (Shain & Groeneveld, 1980; Berger, 1983). Warner-Lambert Canada estimated a return of about $8.50 per dollar spent—80% was attributable to reduced absenteeism, and 20% was attributable to group insurance savings and less frequent accidents.

Illinois Bell claimed a 10:1 return on investment; the proportion of those receiving assistance who were rated as good employees rose from 10% to 46% in the men, and 22% to 58% in the women.

The Philadelphia police department found a 30% reduction of absenteeism and a 62% decrease of injury days after introduction of an employee assistance program.

Productivity

Productivity is often outside the control of the individual worker. Output may be restricted by poor management, delay in the delivery of materials, antiquated machinery, breakdown of equipment, absenteeism of colleagues, lack of market demand for products, seasonal factors, or union restrictions upon performance. However, physical training can improve the output of employees who operate at high fractions of aerobic power or muscular strength (Laporte, 1966; Shephard, 1977b). In mental tasks, physical training may also relieve boredom or stress and improve vigilance. In both physical and mental work, gains of worker satisfaction also may boost productivity (Table 4.1).

Table 4.1 Fitness/Lifestyle Programs and Productivity

Author	Benefit
Rohmert (1973)	Less fatigue, faster recovery
Laporte (1966)	Greater strength, hand steadiness, less eye-fatigue
Pravosudov (1978)	Output standard +2-5% to +10-15%
Réville (1970)	31% decrease of errors
Geissler (1960)	Reduced fatigue
Manguroff, Channe, & Georgieff (1960)	Reduced fatigue
Galevskaya (1970)	Reduced fatigue
Pravosudov (1978)	Greater creativity, less fatigue
Heinzelmann (1975)	Greater self-reported productivity
Howard & Michalachki (1979)	No benefit in middle managers
Finney (1979)	No benefit from recreational programs
Stallings, O'Rourke, & Gross (1975)	No effect on teaching or research output
Blair et al. (1980)	No effect on supervisor assessments, merit pay or promotions
Health & Welfare Canada	4% gain in productivity
Mealey (1979)	39% increase in police-officer commendations
Briggs (1975, February)	Improved memory, muscle control, work performance
Shephard et al. (1981)	2.7% gain in productivity

Physical Work

In physically taxing occupations, muscular weakness increases perceived effort and leads to earlier and more severe fatigue (Rohmert, 1973) and a need for longer recovery pauses. Laporte (1966) noted that provision of an exercise break increased the muscular strength and hand-steadiness of postal workers while it reduced their eye fatigue. In consequence improvements were made in both the quality and the quantity of the work performed.

Kmuzoz (1975) and Pravosudov (1978, p. 262) made cross-sectional comparisons between worker-athletes and sedentary employees in Russian factories. They suggested, apparently from estimates of maximum oxygen intake rather than direct measures of industrial output, that "other things being equal . . . worker athletes had a higher working capacity, . . . their output standard being 2-5% and sometimes 10-15% higher than with nonathletes." They further stated that 5-min exercise breaks were sufficient to improve the coordination of movement and sustain a high level of working activity over a shift and added resultant gains in productivity.

Danielson and Danielson (1982) examined the physical output of forest-fire fighters, expressed as meters of fireline construction per worker-hour. Under relatively easy conditions, the best work was obtained from older, more experienced, but less fit individuals. However, under difficult (hot and dry) conditions a team that received a daily fitness program had twice the productivity of control workers in another sector of the forest.

Mental Work

A spell of physical activity may also improve the quality of work in tasks that require vigilance. Thus Réville (1970) reported a 31% decrease of errors among female textile workers who were given regular exercise breaks. Several authors have commented that when light or sedentary work is required, active gymnastic pauses are more effective than passive pauses in relieving production-line fatigue (Geissler, 1960; Manguroff, Channe, & Georgieff, 1960; Laporte, 1966; Galevskaya, 1970). Stallings, O'Rourke, and Gross (1975) found no correlation between energy expenditure and the academic performance of university faculty, but some suggest that an association may exist between physical and creative activity in Russian scientists (Pravosudov, 1978). Conversely, those who defect from exercise classes have reported a rapid (2-3 week) increase of fatigability (Pravosudov, 1978).

Self-reports that productivity is enhanced by fitness class participation have been noted in the U.S. (Heinzelmann & Bagley, 1970; Durbeck et al., 1972; Heinzelmann, 1975).

Productivity Measurements

In many occupations, obtaining clear, objective measurements of work output is difficult. Perhaps this explains why only a few experiments test the hypothesis that personal fitness enhances productivity (Donoghue, 1977; Haskell & Blair, 1980). Despite the frequent lack of controls and the obvious differences in both the type of employment and the pattern of exercise provided by the company, published results show a fair concordance (Table 4.1).

Howard and Michalachki (1979) noted no increase in the productivity of middle managers after 6 months participation in an employee fitness program. Likewise, Finney (1979) observed little impact of recreational programs upon productivity, while Stallings et al. (1975) found no correlation between sport participation and either the teaching skills or the research output of U.S. faculty. Blair et al. (1980) classified the self-selected leisure activities of 504 white-collar insurance company employees "low," "medium," or "high," corresponding to voluntary energy expenditures of 200, 800, and 2200 kJ • day^{-1}. Activity was unrelated to supervisory assessments, merit pay, or the rate of promotion. However, only 116 of the sample were developing a substantial energy expenditure, and these formed a self-selected group.

In contrast to such negative reports, Carter and Wanzel (1975) maintained that longitudinal studies in both Canada and the U.S. demonstrated favorable effects of employee recreation programs upon fitness, productivity, turnover, absenteeism, and attitudes. Health and Welfare Canada estimated that productivity jumped 4% 1 month after it introduced an exercise break for a group of data processors. The management of the U.S. Xerox Corporation is also of the opinion that productivity at its company has improved since it initiated an employee fitness program (Wanzel, 1979), while Mealey (1979) has commented on a 39% increase in officer commendations in the 6 months following institution of a fitness/lifestyle program for police officers in Dallas. Briggs (1975, February) further claimed that participation in an industrial fitness program improved memory, muscle control, and work performance. Groves (1980) and Groves and DeCarlo (1981) carried out a controlled study of an employee recreation program in a U.S. company; they suggested that job satisfaction was increased in program participants and that they had a productivity gain of 15-25%. Moreover, loss of the recreational opportunities decreased production by 25-35%.

Shephard et al. (1981) carried out a controlled prospective study of life assurance workers in Toronto. Supervisory ratings for such items as promptness of arrival, productivity, accuracy of work, cooperation, and job satisfaction all improved from the preintervention to the experimental year, but changes were rather similar at control and experimental companies. The index of performance applied by management was the integral of the number of hours worked at each of the tasks specified in the individual's job description (calculated from standard times for the performance of these same tasks) divided by the net hours available to the employee (total hours paid minus total hours absent). This method of calculation effectively excludes any benefit from changes in absenteeism. The year following introduction of the employee fitness program, workers at the experimental company showed a 7% rise in this index of productivity. Nevertheless, a part of the gain seems to have been a "Hawthorne" type response because a corresponding estimate of productivity at the control company jumped 4.3%. In this example, the net benefit was a 2.7% relative advantage to the experimental company.

Ascribed Benefit

The gain of productivity seems large enough to merit more careful quantitation. It also has to be established whether the response is exercise specific or is a more general reaction to an improvement in the quality of working life. In support of the latter hypothesis, employees at the Xerox Company fitness program showed an improvement in personal and social self-concept (which presumably accounted for their better productivity), but this change was not clearly related to program attendance or gains in physiological variables such as maximum oxygen intake (Pauly et al., 1982).

Certainly negative reports in the literature suggest that employee fitness programs do not improve productivity in every category of enterprise. Many corporations already operate at less than full capacity for much of the year, and no amount of exercise can correct structural constraints imposed by intransigent management or unions (except indirectly, by fostering good corporate relations). For the purpose of the present analysis, an arbitrary 4% gain of productivity has been ascribed and restricted to active participants in corporate fitness/lifestyle programs. Also, given a 20% program participation rate, the ascribed benefit amounts to 0.8% of payroll (about a third of the effect actually observed in Toronto), or an average annual salary of $14,500, $116 per worker-year. (The effect observed over the first 6 months of the Toronto program amounted to $392 per worker-year.)

Absenteeism

Absenteeism and a high turnover of employees are currently two of the most serious personnel problems facing North American industry (Howard & Michalachki, 1979). In the U.S., the average absenteeism attributable to short-term illness is 3.1 days per year for males and 4.1 days for females (Brennan, 1982a). In Canada, absenteeism probably causes about 11 times the work loss due to strikes (Katz, 1980, September 27). In recent years (Bank of Canada Review, November 1983) strikes have cost from 0.65 days per worker-year (1982) to 1.31 days per worker-year (1976). A recent study from the University of Western Ontario (Ottawa Citizen, 1981, September 28) suggested that only 17% of private companies kept records of sick leave beyond payroll needs. The same report noted that Ontario civil servants each took an average of 10.8 days sick leave per year, and the cost of wages, overtime payments, and replacement staff amounted to $973 per worker-year. One estimate put absenteeism in Canadian industry at 12.7 days per worker-year, for a cost of $977 per employee-year (Industrial Health Assistance, Ltd., 1978). Another report distinguished absenteeism rates of 9.6 days per employee-year in unionized and 5.9 days per employee-year in nonunionized companies. In the U.S., there has been a 25% increase in long-term disabilities from 1966 to 1976 (Wilkins & Adams, 1983), although this may be partly attributable to improved provision for sick employees.

The extent that absenteeism can be modified through improvements of health and fitness is less clear. The Delphic approach of Williamson and Van Nieuwenhuijzen (1974) suggested that about 40% of absenteeism could be reduced by better medical care; the greatest potential for gains was among older workers who were absent 8 or more days per year. Other anecdotal reports suggest that specific fitness/lifestyle programs can reduce absenteeism, particularly absences of 1-2 days, but one must be cautious in inferring a causal relationship between enhanced physical activity and reduced absenteeism. Rather, exercise programs may act through a general improvement in the quality of the working environment.

Fitness and Absenteeism

Lindén (1969) studied cross-sectional correlations between cardiorespiratory fitness and absenteeism among male customs officers, firemen, office workers of both sexes, and miscellaneous employees from other nonsedentary jobs.

The customs officers formed the only occupational group that showed a significant relationship between fitness and absenteeism (coefficient of correlation = 0.47). However, further support for the value of fitness included (a) a low maximum oxygen intake in customs officers and firemen with more than 8 absences per year and (b) a high maximum oxygen intake in office workers with no absenteeism over the year of study.

The main difficulty with Linden's study is the perennial problem of self-selection. Employees who were frequently absent generally came from families of low socioeconomic status, and this in turn influenced various aspects of lifestyle, including both smoking habits and prior participation in voluntary leisure activities.

Fitness Programs and Absenteeism

Popular reports from the U.S. (Condon, 1977, October; Erwin, 1978) suggested that unpaid absenteeism at the People's Credit Jewelers dropped 23% following the institution of an employee fitness program. Likewise, two reports from Romania (Barhad, 1979; Pafnote, Voida, Luchian, 1979) claimed that employee fitness programs reduced absenteeism, although no experimental data were cited. Keelor (1976) indicated to a U.S. governmental committee that absenteeism at the Goodyear Tyre plant in Norkjoping, Sweden, had been halved following introduction of an employee fitness program, while Raab and Gilman (1964) claimed a 68.6% decrease of absenteeism after German workers had spent a month at a Kur resort.

Quantitative reports suggest that the exercise benefit ranges from 0.5 to 5 days per worker year, the magnitude of response depending, in part, upon the initial level of absenteeism (Table 4.2). Pravosudov (1978) noted that Russian worker-athletes consulted a physician four times less often than their sedentary colleagues. Moreover, only 22.5% of consultations by the active workers led to absence from work, whereas 50-60% of the sedentary employees were advised not to report for duty. Benefit was seen in many categories of work, including factories, offices, and the professions, and the advantage to the active group averaged 4 days per worker-year.

Table 4.2 Fitness and Absenteeism—A Summary of Published Reports

Author	Benefit
Lindén (1969)	Correlation of low absenteeism, high $\dot{V}O_2$max
Condon (1978)	23% decrease in absenteeism
Barhad (1979)	Decrease in absenteeism
Pafnote et al. (1979)	Decrease in absenteeism
Keelor (1970)	50% decrease in absenteeism
Pravosudov (1978)	Decrease 4.0 days per worker-year
Mealey (1979)	Decrease of 34% (1.4 days per worker-year)
Wilbur (1983)	Decrease of 22%
Bjurstrom & Alexiou (1978)	Decrease of 0.59 days per worker-year
Blair et al. (1980)	No effect
Richardson (1974, May/June)	Decrease of 0.82 days per worker-year
Garson (1977)	Decrease of 47% (2.8 days per worker-year)
Cox et al. (1981)	Decrease of 23% (1.3 days per worker-year)

Mean of percentage changes: 33%
Mean decrease of absences: 1.8 days per worker-year

The New York Telephone Company estimated annual savings equivalent to more than $3 million from reduced absenteeism and medical treatment costs following introduction of its wellness program (an annual benefit of more than $400 per employee relative to workers in other divisions who did not have access to such a program). In the Dallas police force (Byrd, 1976, December; Mealey, 1979) a 6-month fitness program cut the sick leave of experimental subjects by 29%, while that of control subjects increased by 5%. The program effect was thus 34%, or 1.4 days per worker-year. A preliminary (1-year) report from Johnson and Johnson (C. Wilbur—personal communication) found a 9% decrease in sick days for participants in their lifestyle programs compared with a 13% increase among control employees (net benefit 22%). Bjurstrom and Alexiou (1978) found that 40% of New York State Board of Education workers who joined an employee fitness program decreased their absenteeism; the average effect amounted to 0.59 days per employee-year. The one negative report from the U.S. (Blair et al., 1980) has already been discussed.

Richardson (1974, May/June) observed that recruits in a fitness program at the Canadian post office (headquarters building) initially showed 1.08 days • yr^{-1} less absenteeism than nonparticipants. Over the next year, the advantage of the program participants increased to 1.90 days • yr^{-1} (an apparent exercise benefit of at least 0.82 days • yr^{-1}). In the Metropolitan Life Insurance program (Garson, 1977), participants decreased their absenteeism by 22% (to 4.9 days • yr^{-1}) while nonparticipants showed a 25% increment (to 7.0 days per year). The net program benefit was thus 2.8 days • yr^{-1} (47%).

Typically, it has been necessary to compare participants with non-participants because studies have been conducted largely by occupational medical officers, and employee organizations have shown a reluctance to accept true controlled experiments. However, Cox et al. (1981) were able to compare the absenteeism experience of two rather similar major life assurance company offices for the years 1976/77 and 1977/78 (Table 4.2). At the control company the only forms of intervention were (a) three opportunities for free laboratory fitness tests in 1977/78 and (b) the promise of a fitness program at some future date. Unfortunately, data analysis was complicated by an influenza epidemic in the fall of 1977. At the experimental company, results subsequent to introduction of the employee fitness program (February to June 1978) showed a decline of absenteeism in both experimental and control groups. Classifying the experimental subjects by their interest in the program, high adherents showed a 41.8% decrease in absenteeism. On a simple Chi^2 analysis, this represented a significant advantage relative to both controls (20.1% benefit, $p < 0.01$) and other employees at the experimental company (23.2% benefit, $p < 0.001$). Analysis of variance, using each subject as his or her own control, revealed a similar trend, although intercategory differences were no longer statistically significant. The benefit observed among active participants in this study (1.3 days per person-year) reflects a relatively low overall rate of absenteeism prior to the intervention. Both of the assurance companies involved in the experiment were nonunionized and had a good record of labor relations extending over many years. The benefit to a company with a poor initial attendance record has yet to be explored, although potential would exist for a larger response.

A more detailed analysis of the Toronto Life Assurance Company data showed similar changes in both uncertified and medically certified absences, with no particular impact upon Monday or Friday absences. However, a greater improvement in men than in women was suggested (Cox et al., 1981). A multiple regression analysis (Cox, Shephard, & Corey, 1983) established the dependence of reduced absenteeism upon changes in both aerobic power ($\dot{V}O_2$max ml • $kg^{-1}min^{-1}$) and job satisfaction (work scale of job description index, JDI units):

$$\Delta \text{ absenteeism} = -0.84 \, \Delta\dot{V}O_2\text{max}$$
$$- 0.72 \, \Delta\text{JDI} + 0.12 \, (\Delta\dot{V}O_2\text{max} \cdot \text{JDI})(\text{days} \cdot yr^{-1})$$

The implication of this equation is that the employee fitness program had some independent effect, but the response was smaller in those subjects who also showed a substantial improvement in job satisfaction.

Table 4.3 Absenteeism Rate Before and During an Employee Fitness/Lifestyle Program

| Subject Category | Absenteeism (days • yr⁻¹) | | | |
	Before Program	During Program	Difference	Change (%)
Test company				
High adherents (n = 171)	7.24	4.21	−3.03	−41.8
Low adherents (n = 140)	7.88	7.20	−0.68	−8.7
Dropouts (n = 124)	9.10	9.38	+0.28	+3.1
Nonparticipants (n = 200)	8.22	6.30	−1.92	−23.4
Test company minus high				
adherents (n = 1,110)	8.53	6.86	−1.67	−19.5
Control company (n = 577)	10.13	7.93	−2.20	−21.7

Note. From "Influence of an Employee Fitness Programme Upon Fitness, Productivity and Absenteeism" by M. Cox, R.J. Shephard, and P. Corey, 1981, *Ergonomics*, **24**, pp. 795-806.

Further evidence for a causal component to the relationship between fitness and absenteeism was obtained when observations were repeated after 18 months of the fitness program's operation (Song, Shephard, & Cox, 1982). At this stage, the absenteeism of initial high adherents did not differ from figures for the remainder of the company, but when subjects were reclassified according to their current exercise behavior, an association again was present between class participation and low absenteeism rates.

Ascribed Benefits

The Toronto Life Assurance estimate (1.3 days • yr⁻¹ decrease of absenteeism in high adherents to the fitness/lifestyle program) may well be a conservative measure of benefit in view of the low initial absenteeism rates at the two companies studied.

Assuming a replacement cost of 1.75 times lost time (chapter 1) with 20% of employees becoming high adherents to the program, 220 working days per year, and a salary of $14,500 per annum, the savings from the fitness program would amount to (1.75 × 1.3/220 × 20/100 × 14,500), or $30 per worker-year. To the extent that higher-paid (older and more senior) workers become high adherents, this figure is an underestimate of the program-related benefit.

A need plainly exists to study the impact of exercise programs on companies that initially have a high absenteeism rate. It would also be interesting to compare responses between programs that induce large gains in fitness indices such as $\dot{V}O_2$(max) and others that emphasize an improvement in the quality of working life instead.

Turnover

The economic importance of turnover depends upon the availability of labor and the costs of training. For some production-line tasks, a turnover rate of 50% per annum may not have serious economic repercussions except insofar as it indicates that the workers are dissatisfied and may therefore produce goods of poor quality. At the opposite extreme, some companies set a replacement value of $0.5-1.0M upon their senior executives (Donoghue, 1977).

If turnover is very high (e.g., 50% per year) it can have a major impact upon program effectiveness. Employees who are about to give notice are unlikely to join an exercise class, while new recruits are not part of established social networks, and thus may miss key promotional information. Furthermore, even if exercise habits are initiated, such behavior is likely to be lost once an employee leaves the company, and in any event the company will not benefit from long-term improvements in health (Kristein, 1982).

Effect of Exercise

The initial turnover rate in the Toronto Life Assurance study (18% per annum) was lower than in many blue-collar industries, which indicates above-average baseline work satisfaction (Cox et al., 1981). Nevertheless, both low and high adherents to the exercise program showed less subsequent turnover than did nonparticipants or dropouts. Indeed, program participants had a turnover rate of only 1.8% per annum subsequent to initiation of the project.

Wilson (1982) had similar findings in a study of British Columbia Hydro employees; the turnover of fitness program participants was 3.5%, as compared with the divisional average of 10.3%.

Turnover is essentially a once-only event, and the behavior of an individual thus cannot be followed prospectively. Self-selection of a satisfied group of workers cannot be ruled out as one possible explanation of either the Toronto or the British Columbia data. However, retrospective questioning does not suggest that the high adherents in the Toronto study were an inherently stable group of employees (Table 4.4). The average initial duration of service was 8.3 years for controls, 11.3 years for nonparticipants, 9.8 years for dropouts, 8.1 years for low adherents, and

Table 4.4 Initial Estimates of Turnover Rate for Toronto Life Assurance Study

Subject Group	Average Duration of Service (yr)	Estimated* < 1 yr of Service (%)	Actual < 1 yr of Service (%)	Estimated† Turnover Rate (%)
Controls	8.3	6.02	—	12.0
Nonparticipants	11.3	4.42	6.00	8.9
Dropouts	9.8	5.10	8.06	10.2
Low adherents	8.1	6.17	2.86	12.3
High adherents	9.7	5.15	5.84	10.3

*Calculated as (2/average duration of service)100.

†Calculated as (1/average duration of service)100.

Note. Calculated from reported duration of service. From "Influence of an Employee Fitness Programme Upon Fitness, Productivity and Absenteeism" by M. Cox, R.J. Shephard, and P. Corey, 1981, *Ergonomics,* **24**, pp. 795-806.

9.7 years for high adherents. It did not appear that any of these averages were biased greatly by subjects with very high turnover rates. The turnover estimated from a simple inversion* of these various numbers (8.8-12.3%) is a little lower than that currently observed for the entire experimental company; nevertheless, the average (9.6 years, 7.0%) coincides closely with the initial (preexperimental) figure for high adherents and argues against the selection of stable employees into the exercise program.

It may thus be inferred that the 16.2% reduction of annual turnover in activity class adherents is a program benefit, although further study would be necessary to be sure that it was related to a gain of fitness rather than to some other change of lifestyle initiated by the project.

Ascribed Benefit

At the Toronto Life Assurance companies, the cost of hiring and training a new employee is estimated at $13,600 for executives and $6400 for clerical personnel. Savings would depend upon (a) the relative numbers of executives and clerical personnel, (b) their relative participation in the fitness/lifestyle program, and (c) their relative susceptibility to a change of turnover rate. This information is not presently available, and we have

---

Note. Actuarial tables cannot be used because long-standing employees make a disproportionate contribution to the average longevity.

made the simplifying assumption of a uniform cost of $10,000 per replacement.

Assuming also an exercise participation rate of 20%, the annual savings would amount to ($10,000 × 16.2/100 × 20/100), or $324 per worker-year. Scope remains to carry out more precise calculations on groups differing in both turnover rate and cost of replacement.

Another notable observation is that in some companies the existence of a fitness/lifestyle program facilitates recruitment, so the cost of replacing a worker diminishes. In the same context, the program may have a favorable impact upon public perceptions of a company, particularly if the product that is marketed is health-related (e.g., insurance, pharmaceuticals, food, or soft drinks). Corporate investment in image-making is at best an imprecise science, and no attempt is made here to ascribe a dollar value to such activity.

Injuries

Some industrial injuries arise from external trauma and from psychoneurosis. Exercise could conceivably help reduce such statistics by increasing vigilance and/or decreasing alcohol and drug abuse. Internal trauma, usually affecting the spine, is a more common industrial problem. Contributory factors on the part of the employee include poor posture, obesity, lack of physical fitness, and faulty techniques when lifting or carrying heavy loads (C.I.S., 1962; Guthrie, 1963). Enhanced physical activity could reduce the incidence of such accidents.

Current Cost of Industrial Injuries

Brown (1972) reported that back injuries cost the Province of Ontario the equivalent of $19.4M per annum (about $9 per worker-year). More recent estimates suggest a substantially larger total cost for industrial injuries. Thus in 1974, 1400 Canadian hospital beds were occupied by work-related injuries, and work-related deaths totaled 1465 (1 per 6000 worker-years). The compensable injury rate was 0.1145 per worker-year. Average claims were the equivalent of $1120 (an expense of $128.24 per worker-year), and further indirect costs (loss of productivity, material damage, and industrial retraining) were equivalent to $451.35 per worker-year (Chisholm, 1977). In 1976, Canada again sustained 927 work-related fatalities, and total payments were equivalent to $1.5B for injuries and illnesses (World Health Forum, 1981).

In the U.S., which has about 10 times the Canadian population, accidents led to 245 million lost workdays in 1979 (U.S. National Safety Council, 1980). About 200 million of the annual lost workdays in the U.S. are attributable to back injuries (Goldberg, Cohn, Dehn, & Seeds, 1980, June); 50% of the workers experience significant back pain at some point in their careers (Andrevsky, 1982, December).

In Ontario, the most common type of lesion is a sacroiliac strain (82% of claims, average disability 28 days). An additional 12% of workers develop visceral hernias, while 6% of claims relate to slipped intervertebral discs. This last category of injury has the greatest industrial importance because the period of disability is long (average 135 days), and alternative employment often needs to be arranged for the affected individual.

Impact of Exercise Programs

The importance of regular physical activity to avoid back injuries is suggested by the fact that such internal trauma is more common in occupations in which lifting is not a regular occurrence. Likewise, the supervisor may be more vulnerable than the average employee who maintains his or her physical condition by lifting every day (Guthrie, 1963; Shephard, 1974).

Pravosudov (1978) claimed that "professional traumatism" was 2-10 times less frequent in workers who took up physical training than in those who did not. However, self-selection may have discouraged those with incipient back pain from sport participation. Mealey (1979) noted a high incidence of lower-back problems, pulled muscles, and strained ankles and wrists in the Dallas police force. Such problems became less frequent in a group that participated in a 6-month fitness program. Likewise, Superko, Bernauer, and Voss (1983) found that the injury experience of Californian police improved after an 18-month fitness program. Back dysfunction decreased from 0.61 to 0.13% of the force, injuries requiring medical evaluation dropped from 1.16 to 0.32%, and the proportion of officers who passed an aerobic fitness test increased from 59.2 to 68.4%. Results of a longitudinal (but uncontrolled) study of the Los Angeles Fire Department suggested that over 3 years an employee fitness program saved 3725 injury-days at an estimated value of about $483,000 (Barnard & Anthony, 1980).

Scope remains for a carefully controlled prospective study of the impact of fitness/lifestyle programs on the risk of intercurrent injuries both at work and at home. Such an investigation should include statistics on injuries caused by exercise programs and should cover both blue- and white-collar occupations.

Ascribed Benefit

If we accept the as yet unconfirmed view of Pravosudov (1978), an employee fitness program could reduce injuries by 50-90%. While little or no savings would show up in white-collar work, the benefit from injury reduction need not be discounted because the originally cited cost of such disabilities ($128.24 direct and $451.35 indirect per worker-year) was distributed over the entire labor force.

Absenteeism has already been considered, and the indirect costs of injury should possibly be adjusted downward to discount this item. Nevertheless, in some investigations such as the Toronto Life Assurance study, few industrial injuries were initially present, so the experimental program had little opportunity to demonstrate its potential for controlling the injury component of absenteeism. Assuming a labor cost of $14,500/220 ($66 • day^{-1}) and setting the loss of productivity at 1.75 times this figure ($116 per day), the 11.5M annual days of work loss due to injury would cost $1.33B, or $151.76 per worker-year. The allowable portion of the indirect cost is thus ($451.35 − $151.76), or $299.59 per worker-year.

Of the direct costs, hospital care has been considered elsewhere (chapter 2). However, the program impact was calculated for a company in which no significant industrial injuries existed. Thus the hospital cost of $81.8M ($9.30 per worker-year) need not be deducted. The allowable cost of industrial injury is ($128.24 + $299.59), or $427.83 per worker-year.

Taking the most conservative of Pravosudov's estimates (50% reduction) and assuming an equal impact upon minor, major, and fatal injuries, with 20% program participation the ascribed benefit would amount to ($427.83 × 0.5 × 0.2), or $42.78 per worker-year. This figure must be viewed with some caution though, because a major component is the indirect cost of premature death, and it is not yet clear whether fatal industrial accidents would be materially reduced by a fitness/lifestyle program.

Conclusions

The total fiscal benefit to a company from an employee fitness program (Table 4.5) may be estimated at $513 per worker-year. In principle, the benefit is realized whether the program is company- or community-based, but in the latter situation lower participation rates tend to reduce savings. The main elements in the cost-benefit calculations are turnover costs (which vary widely from one company to another) and potential gains of productivity. Although not formally costed, the higher quality of production associated with improved worker satisfaction may also boost sales and reduce the expense of warranty work. Moreover, if supplemen-

Table 4.5 Summary of Industrial Benefits From Fitness/Lifestyle Programs

Benefit	Fiscal Saving
Employment in fitness services	Labor-intensive
Worker satisfaction	Higher quality production—less warranty work
Productivity	$116 per worker-year
Absenteeism	$ 30 per worker-year
Turnover	$324 per worker-year
Industrial injury	$ 43 per worker-year
Health insurance premiums	Reduced (?32%)
Company image	Enhanced by in-house program
Total	$513 per worker-year

tary health insurance is purchased for employees, negotiating a reduction of premiums of up to 32% could be possible, based on the information given in chapter 2.

No mandatory entries exist on the debit side of the ledger unless physical activity is pursued to the point of producing fatigue and musculoskeletal injuries. Many companies now believe that the benefits of physical activity are sufficiently well-established, and they are investing in corporate fitness/lifestyle programs. The cost varies with the luxury of facilities and the completeness of accounting. Some U.S. corporations charge their fitness divisions high rentals for space and occupancy. Wanzel (1979) estimated the Canadian cost at $100-$350 per participant year, or with an anticipated participation rate of 20%, $20-$70 per worker-year, which works out to be 4-14% of the anticipated fiscal benefit to the company.

chapter 5

Geriatric Consequences
of Enhanced Physical Fitness

Historically, the hospice was a place for travelers to rest during a jour-
ney. The name has currently been adopted by a movement in our western
culture which seeks care for the person resting along the journey of life
toward death. (Goodell, 1985, p. 960)

Senior citizens impose a substantial charge upon the national economy partly because they are dependent members of society and partly because they consume a substantial fraction of acute and chronic medical care resources. Some suggest that medical and hospital costs per individual are five times larger for those who exceed 65 years of age. The geriatric burden will increase further in many nations as the population ages, but an enhancement of personal fitness could make a substantial contribution to the containment of such costs.

Actuarial Considerations and Retirement Policy

Dependency Costs

In its simplest form, the dependency ratio D is given by

$$D = (C + E)/A$$

where C is the number of children, E is the number of elderly, and A is the number of working-age adults. Data are sometimes cited for the aged dependency ratio (E/A), and a need also exists to calculate statistics for the "very old" (E'/A) because they are likely to be the most costly members of society. Some projections indicate a doubling in the proportion of "very old" citizens over the next 30 years (Paillat, 1977; Lipman, 1979).

The standard dependency ratio depends on (a) the birth rate over the previous 14-18 years, (b) the average age when a child leaves school (14 years according to Paillat, 1971, but 17 years according to Decker, 1980, and 19 years according to Denton & Spencer, 1980a), (c) the proportion of unemployed young adults (currently high and increasing), (d) net migration, (e) the age of retirement (assumed to be 65 years in many calculations), and (f) the number of senior citizens (likely to increase substantially over the next 2 decades).

In the U.S., the dependency ratio was 0.64 in 1950, but increased to 0.82 in 1960 (due to the baby boom). By 1976 it had dropped back to 0.69 (Decker, 1980). However, the old age dependency ratio rose from 0.13 in 1950 to 0.17 in 1960 and 0.18 in 1976 and had a predicted value of 0.32 by the year 2030. Denton and Spencer (1980a) cited a total Canadian dependency ratio of 0.80 in 1976 with an old-age dependency ratio of 0.16; the latter is expected to reach 0.33 by the year 2031.

More refined economic calculations take account of the differing material needs of children, working adults, and the retired elderly. Paillat (1971) set the needs of French children and senior citizens at 70% of the figure for active adults, and calculated on this basis that a proportion P of active individuals' earnings would be needed to finance pension funds, such that

$$P = \frac{0.7E}{0.7(C + E) + A + A'}$$

where E was the number of senior citizens, C was the number of children and full-time students, A was the number of active adults, and A' was the number of adults not participating in the work force (the unemployed, homemakers, etc.). In 12 European countries, pensions actually averaged only 33.1% of working salaries (28.6-36.5%) and had a corresponding P value of 7.3% (range 5.4-9.0%). It was further estimated that a 50% pension for all senior citizens would require an increase of P to 11.2%, while a 75% pension would necessitate a P of 16.8%. Because of a more favorable age pyramid, current Canadian values of P are a little lower for any given pension rate; but if present demographic trends continue, European levels may be reached over the next 2-3 decades.

Applying Paillat's formula to Canadian population statistics, P lies in the range 8.63-9.51%, given a 70% fiscal provision for retirees. Costs in North America exceed this simple estimate because (a) almost all children continue their schooling to 18 rather than 14 years, (b) up to 20% of young adults remain as partial dependents to 22 years of age, and (c) the proportion of institutionalized elderly is higher in North America than

in Europe. Using comparable age break points, a more appropriate formula for North American society might be

$$P = \frac{0.78E}{0.78E + 0.95C + A + A'}$$

with P values in the range 8.98-9.96%.

The current governmental pension plan in Canada provides $5484
per annum to a single retiree and $7620 per annum to a married couple.
Given gross earnings of $14,500 per annum, these figures amount to 45%
and 58% of disposable preretirement income (gross income less federal
and provincial taxes). On average, a little less than half of senior citizens'
income is derived from governmental schemes (Powell & Martin, 1980).
In 1975, 22% of elderly couples and 61% of elderly singles (mostly women)
lived below the official poverty line and spent more than 70% of their
incomes on listed "necessities" of life.

The proportion of money allocated to pensions is ultimately a political decision, and as the number of senior citizens rises, they will have
an increasing impact upon the electoral process (Pratt, 1976; Hudson &
Binstock, 1976), particularly because they are more likely than young
people to exercise their franchise (Sheppard, 1971; Shephard & LaBarre,
1978; Glenn & Grimes, 1968).

Age of Retirement

Physical activity could reduce dependency costs if it postponed the
normal age of retirement. Variables influencing the decision to retire include legislation, financial security, work satisfaction, and the demand
for labor in addition to the physical and mental health of the employee.

Human rights legislators are just beginning to examine the question
of mandatory retirement. Some states and provinces currently proscribe
age discrimination in employment (Chappell, 1980), and it seems likely
that in the future employees will be allowed to remain in most occupations as long as they remain competent and meet minimum standards
of physical health specific to their tasks. Thus U.S. federal legislation has
prohibited age discrimination in employment since 1967, and in 1978 the
ceiling of this protection was raised from 64 to 70 years, exceptions being
allowed for a few specific categories of worker such as business executives, air-traffic controllers, law-enforcement officers, and firefighters.

Fears of inflation and a knowledge that many senior citizens currently
live in poverty are important pressures holding older people in the work
force. Given an adequately indexed pension plan, Shaver and Tobin (1978)

found that a majority of pilots and white- and blue-collar employees of a U.S. airline would choose to retire at 55 rather than 65 years of age. A further important factor is the nature of the work performed. Intellectuals are reluctant to abandon a job that they enjoy (Antonini, 1971; Shanas, 1971; Friedmann & Orbach, 1974), but "the only deterrent to people retiring from a factory is whether they will be able to live . . . in the mode or manner in which they have become accustomed" (Shanas, 1971, p. 117). While 86% of U.S. citizens agreed with the statement "Nobody should be forced to retire because of age if he wants to continue working and is still able to do a good job" (Decker, 1980), 61% of U.S. citizens over the age of 65 years reported that they had retired voluntarily.

Early retirement is sometimes regarded as having social value because it augments employment opportunities for the young (Back, 1969; Sauvy, 1970; Parker, Thomas, Ellis, & McCarthy, 1971). This factor depends upon the growth of robotics relative to compensatory development of service industries. From current projections, the need for elderly workers to continue in most occupations may be decreasing (Tindale & Marshall, 1980). On the other hand, continued employment of older workers sometimes has a profound influence upon the overall structure and ambience of a corporation by improving organizational effectiveness and encouraging the retention of younger employees (Schrank & Riley, 1978).

Physical prospects for continuing employment depend upon socioeconomic status, the level of training and experience that has been accumulated, physical health, emotional stability, in some occupations physical stamina, potential for job redesign (Adachi, 1978; Andrisani, 1978), and opportunities for retraining within a company (Montgomery, 1978).

Adaptation to Retirement

The process of retirement involves a major change in many facets of lifestyle (Howard, Marshall, Rechnitzer, Cunningham, & Donner, 1982), and regular physical activity may play an important role in facilitating such adaptation.

Friedman and Havighurst (1954) suggested that retirement caused a sense of loss for the individual. Absence of regular work robbed the senior citizen of both norms of behavior and a means of integrating into society. Some authors argue that the constructive use of leisure can restore personal identity and meaning (Atchley, 1971), although others point out that no form of imposed leisure can provide the same sense of self-respect as a job (Miller, 1965).

Retirement involves a process of accommodation as time and energy are redistributed (Shanas, 1971). Financial resources play a significant role in facilitating adjustment, but the pursuit of active leisure is a critical determinant of adaptation to retirement (Darnley, 1975; DeCarlo, 1974) and subsequent life satisfaction (Draper, 1967).

Successful adaptation to retirement is, in part, an opportunity dividend of enhanced physical activity and as such is difficult to quantitate. However, to the extent that new interests avert depression and restore failing cognitive functions, real dollar savings are also available in both acute and chronic health care costs.

Ascribed Benefit

Physical activity could curtail the period of dependency through effects on health, stamina, and mental functioning. Beverfeldt (1971) commented that 40% of Norwegian retirees who wanted to work and 60% of those who did not were medically incapable of carrying out their occupations. Likewise, results of a survey from the U.K. showed that 30-35% of manual workers and 23% of nonmanual workers were in poor health by the age of 65 years (Richardson, 1964). However, much if not all of the potential benefit from an activity-induced improvement of health has already been considered under such headings as a reduction in "appraised age" (chapter 2).

The sign of a loss of physical stamina is a decrease in maximum oxygen intake, which amounts to about 0.5 ml/kg • min per year (Shephard, 1978). Vigorous physical activity does not alter the rate of this loss in those who are already well-trained, but it does improve the functional age of the average senior citizen by the equivalent of at least 8 years (a gain in oxygen transport of about 4-5 ml/kg • min (Shephard, 1978b; Süominen, Heikkinen, Parkatte, Forsberg, & Kiiskinen, 1977; Borkan & Norris, 1980). Scope is available to ascertain exactly how many senior citizens are encountering physical limitations in their working abilities at retirement. However, a reasonable operating assumption is that no more than 10% of the present population are engaged in such heavy work that a gain in stamina would materially extend their working spans. The possible bogey is that if the health of the senior citizen were improved, pensions would also be paid over a longer span (Gori & Richter, 1978). If the quality of retired life were also enhanced, this would be a worthwhile expense. But at present no evidence proves that exercise would extend longevity. Thus if 20% of heavy manual workers were persuaded to participate in a fitness/lifestyle program, the benefit from an extension of employed years would amount to $14,500 × 10/100 × 20/100, or $290 per year. Distributing an 8-year benefit over a working career of 40 years, the maximum gain would be $58 per worker-year.

Not all of the potential benefit would necessarily be realized. While a person sometimes encounters problems with paced work in his or her late 40s (Fulgraff, 1971), an unfit employee may compensate for waning physical powers through (a) experience and skill, (b) task delegation by virtue of seniority, and (c) operation at a slower pace. Moreover, in many occupations the limiting factor is no longer physical stamina, but rather the ability to adapt to the demands of new machinery (Chown, 1962; Eisdorfer, 1969).

Medical Care of the Elderly

Institutionalized care for the elderly currently imposes a total burden of about $3820M per year upon Canadian society ($2247 per senior citizen). A somewhat similar figure can be calculated for the U.S. (Tables 5.1 and 5.2). The relative cost of acute and chronic care hospitals and

Table 5.1 Approximate Costs of Institutional Care for the Elderly*

Type of Care	Percent of Elderly Population	Population in Canada	Daily Costs˟ ($)	Annual Costs ($)
Active treatment	1.47	24,990	222	2,025M
Chronic treatment	0.89	15,130	61	337M
Mental care	0.32	5,440	61	121M
Extended care	4.17	70,890	34	880M
Other residential care	2.30	39,100	32†	457M
Total			410	3,820M

*Data for the city of London, Ontario, upgraded to 1983 Canadian dollars. Capital cost of facilities *not* included. For simplicity, calculations have been based upon changes in the Consumer Price Index. In fact, the costs of institutional care have tended to outstrip the CPI over this period, while the proportion of senior citizens has also increased; the cost of $3,820M is thus best expressed as $2,247 per senior citizen per year.

†Includes a charge of $20 per day for occupation of ambulatory care residence and an amount that varies with the amount of nursing care that is required.

˟The latest figures from Statistics Canada show even higher costs (acute care $241, rehabilitation $214, chronic care $105, and extended care $105); this reflects in part the fact that hospital costs have substantially outpaced the CPI.

Note. From "Responses of Elderly Subjects to Training," doctoral dissertation by K.H. Sidney, 1975, Toronto: University of Toronto.

Table 5.2 Annual Cost of Health Care for Elderly Citizens in the U.S.*

Cost	Amount ($M)
Hospital care	1,212
Physicians' services	444
Other professional services	105
Drugs	273
Nursing home care	420
Miscellaneous	120
Total	$2,574

*From U.S. Senate Report, 1972, but updated to 1983 Canadian dollars. For simplicity, the overall Consumer Price Index has been used in adjusting costs. In fact, medical costs have outstripped the CPI over this period.

residential homes in the U.K. conforms to the North American pattern (a ratio of 6:2:1; Ross, 1978).

Further study of factors leading to institutionalization is needed. Wilson and Levy (1978) found that 34% of the admissions to a Scottish geriatric unit had acute physical illnesses and 11% had acute mental illnesses, but in the remainder, the decision was based upon chronic physical disease, difficult nursing, and inadequate family support. Brocklehurst (1973) noted that social factors played a major role in admission. On the average, almost twice as many senior citizens are institutionalized in the U.S. and Canada as in the U.K. (Schwenger & Gross, 1980), and there are also marked regional differences (Wilkins & Adams, 1983). Major handicaps to those living on the North American continent include greater dispersion of the family and difficulty in finding a physician who is willing to make housecalls (Groth-Junker, 1983, March 22). If a home health-care team is available, medical costs for the elderly can be reduced by 8.6%. Moreover, individuals treated by the home care team spend 38% fewer days in hospitals and 58% fewer days in nursing homes, while the proportion dying at home, initially 47%, is increased to 71%.

Groth-Junker (1983) noted the five most frequent medical problems of the elderly as cancer, stroke, arthritis/rheumatism, dementia, and arteriosclerotic heart disease. Diagnoses on admission to a British institution are summarized in Table 5.3. At the acute treatment center, the main problems were cardiovascular diseases and strokes, while in the geriatric unit chronic brain syndrome was the prime disorder. Statistics on the causes of death for senior citizens follow a similar general pattern

Table 5.3 Admission Diagnoses of Elderly Patients Entering Acute Treatment Center (Internal Medical Department) and Chronic Treatment Center (Geriatric Unit)

Cause of Admission	Acute Treatment Center %	Chronic Treatment Center %	%*
Cardiovascular disease	42	24	34
Stroke	22	13	18
Chronic respiratory disease	8	16	22
Acute infection	11	11	15
Chronic brain syndrome	0	28	—
Coma	0	3	4
Other	17	5	7
Total	100	100	100

*Assuming chronic brain syndrome treated in an institution for mental disorders.

Note. From "Geriatric Services and the Day Hospital" by J.C. Brocklehurst, 1973. In J.C. Brocklehurst (Ed.), *Textbook of Geriatric Medicine and Gerontology* (p. 676), Edinburgh: Churchill-Livingstone.

Table 5.4 Leading Causes of Death in U.S. Senior Citizens

Condition	Percent of Deaths Age > 65 yr
Cardiac diseases	46
Cancer	15
Cerebrovascular diseases	15
Influenza and pneumonia	4
Arteriosclerosis	3
Accidents	2
Diabetes mellitus	2
Bronchitis/emphysema/asthma	2
Other	11

Note. From "Health in the later years of life" by the National Center for Health Statistics, 1971, Washington, DC: U.S. Government Printing Office, cited in *Social Gerontology* (p. 61) by D.L. Decker, 1980, Boston: Little, Brown.

(Table 5.4). At an acute treatment center, the main causes of death were cardiovascular (32%), cancerous (27%), digestive (13%), respiratory (12%), and nervous (9%), while at the geriatric unit cardiac and respiratory deaths were dominant (Timaras, 1972). Brocklehurst (1973) noted that 74% of acute patients were discharged, 22% died, and 4% stayed in the hospital more than 3 months. In contrast, 29% of geriatric patients were discharged, 33% died, and 38% (presumably mainly the senile dementias) remained in the hospital.

Data from the Canada Health Survey (1982) suggest an average expectation (at birth) of 10.8 years of restricted activity in men and 14.0 years in women, followed by 0.8 or 1.5 years of institutionalization (Wilkins & Adams, 1983). Annual disability days rise from an average of 15.7 in men and 12.5 in women of all ages to 35.0 and 30.2 in men and women aged 65 years or older. In U.S. senior citizens, a potential of 8.3 years of restricted activity and 0.9 years of institutional care remain (Goldschmidt, unpublished data, 1983).

About a half of deaths in people over the age of 65 years are attributable to cardiac or cerebrovascular disease (Lalonde, 1974). In men, lung cancer, chronic chest disease, and other cancers account for a further sixth of deaths, while in women, various types of cancer account for about one sixteenth of deaths.

Potential Savings

The prime categories of disorder requiring acute treatment (cardiovascular disease, stroke/hypertension, chronic respiratory disease) are all conditions in which exercise has some potential benefit. It has been argued that the extent of savings is likely to be less in the elderly than in younger individuals because pathological changes (myocardial degeneration, emphysema) become irreversible at this stage. However, the real factor governing admission to an institution is usually not the medical condition, but rather the ability of the patient to cope with the activities of daily living, and in this context physical status may be quite important. Further data are needed, but for the present it is assumed that the outcome of participation in an endurance exercise program will be a 25% reduction in admissions for cardiovascular disease and a 10% reduction in stroke and chronic respiratory disease admissions—this reflects the not unrealistic supposition that the cardiovascular benefit is at least a half of that anticipated in younger age groups and that some benefit (about 10%) still accrues from the reduction of blood pressure (strokes) and prevention of muscle wasting (chronic respiratory disease). The composite overall decrease in admissions for acute treatment then becomes 13.5% (Table 5.5).

Chronic Treatment. Canadian statistics treat mental disorders separately from other chronic disorders. The other diagnostic categories are similar to those noted for acute admissions. Weighting the savings from a physical activity program in similar fashion to the weighting adopted for acute

Table 5.5 Potential Reduction in Costs of Geriatric Institutional Care Resulting From an Increase in Physical Activity Among the Elderly

Type of Care	Annual Cost ($)	Saving Factor	Dollar Savings ($)
Active treatment	2,025M	0.135	273M
Chronic treatment	337M	0.125	42M
Mental care	121M	0.10	12M
Extended care	880M	0.67	713M
Other residential care	457M	0.67	306M
Total			$1,346M

Notes. Saving of $1346M is equivalent to $792 per senior citizen per year. If work span = 40 years, retirement span = 12 years, saving = $238 per worker-year, or given a program impact of 20%, $48 per worker-year. If active and chronic treatment items are allowed elsewhere, net savings are $606 per senior citizen-year or $182 per worker-year; with a program impact of 20%, this yields $36.40 per worker-year.

Data from Table 5.1.

disorders, a 12.5% overall decrease in admissions for chronic treatment is found.

Mental Care. No reliable information seems to be available on how the incidence of senile dementia might be affected by regular physical activity. Because the mental problem arises from a combination of cerebral atherosclerosis and hypertensive hemorrhage, it would seem acceptable to impute some advantage to exercise (atherosclerosis is lessened, resting blood pressure is reduced about 5 mmHg, and the exercise pressure is also less at a given rate of working). For the purpose of the present calculations, an arbitrary 10% reduction in new admissions has been assumed.

Extended and Residential Care. The most intriguing item in the calculation is a possible reduction in the demand for extended and residential care. Such care is commonly provided because the individual concerned is no longer able to cope with demands of daily living like shopping, cleaning, and keeping house. An improvement of physical condition could thus do much to extend the period of independence or life in a small and inexpensive group home.

A need exists to examine variables limiting independence; loss of flexibility or muscle strength may be more important than a decline in aerobic power. However, the average sedentary person is limited by a maximum oxygen transport of less than $1 \, l \cdot min^{-1}$ at the age of 79 years (Shephard, 1978). A program of vigorous training augments oxygen transport by 20%, and it takes an additional 8-9 years for function to wane to the same limiting level.

About 30% of the population survive to the age of 79 years, but only 10% live to the age of 88 years (Comfort, 1973). Thus if exercise has had no effect upon longevity, an enhancement of physical activity could possibly reduce the number of individuals unable to care for themselves from 30% to 10%. True gains will necessarily be somewhat smaller because the onset of organic pathologies has some bearing upon admissions even to extended-care homes.

Ascribed Benefit

Potential reductions in the costs of geriatric institutional care are summarized in Table 5.5. A large part of the decrease in costs for acute and chronic treatment has already been allowed under personal benefits (chapter 2). The potential for unique savings (related to reduced mental, extended, and residential care) amount to $1031M per year, or $606 per senior citizen per year. Assuming a retirement span of 12 years and a work span of 40 years, the estimated benefit is $36.40 per worker-year with a 20% program impact.

The relatively high cost of providing specialized exercise facilities so that senior citizens may maintain their activity must be set against this benefit.

Conclusions

Enhanced fitness can save society money by extending the span of working life and reducing the period for which institutional support is required. However, a large part of the likely benefit has already been allowed in other sectors of the balance sheet. An apparent need is to disaggregate the savings in order to calculate cost/benefit ratios at various ages. Inevitably, exercise programs for the elderly are costly, but potential medical care savings may also accrue among retirees.

chapter 6

Costs of
Enhanced Physical Fitness

I can foresee a time when squash courts, recreation rooms and swimming pools will become a mandatory and integral part of every major building, whether it be hotel, factory, flat or office block—as usual and necessary as modern plumbing. (Bannister, 1972)

Much of the cost of fitness and recreational facilities currently falls upon municipal governments. For example, the total recreational investment in Ontario for 1983 was estimated at $406M (Berger, 1983); the federal component (0.9% of this total) and the provincial component (3.7%) were mainly for the development of large regional parks, while the private sector investment (66.7%) was concentrated heavily upon theaters and resources for passive amusement. This left the municipal investment (28.7%) to cover local needs for active indoor and outdoor recreational facilities. Many people view leisure time as a period for consumption; they see a dichotomy between production (at work) and consumption (at play), and thus scope may be available to extend the role of the commercial sector beyond its present provision of equipment to an increased involvement in the provision of programs and facilities. Certainly, public sector costs would be less if the family that bought cross-country skis from a sporting goods store did not expect free or low-cost public park facilities to exploit its purchase.

Total municipal spending on recreation in Ontario during 1983 was about $631M $\cdot$ yr^{-1}, or $89 per citizen. About 81.4% of this total represented the operating budget, and 18.6% represented the capital budget. Provincial transfer payments covered 18.7% of the capital expenditures; 23% of operating expenditures were obtained from user fees, and an average of 1.6% were provided by the province (with larger subsidies going to small municipalities, where costs per capita were necessarily greater).

The main source of municipal revenue continues to be the local mill rate (1 mill = 10 cents per $100 rateable value). Given such an arrangement, the available income varies with distribution of the tax base between commercial, industrial, and residential land. In the U.S., a typical recreational allowance is about 12% of municipal revenues (Hjelte & Shivers, 1978). Other possibilities for public sector financing include a specific recreational millage tax, various types of bond issues, federal and state or provincial lotteries, bequests, leaseback arrangements, and income from concessions.

Direct Costs

The main emphasis up to this point has been upon the benefits of physical activity. However, direct costs for exercise testing and prescription, construction and operation of exercise facilities, leadership training, program development, promotion, and the treatment of recreational injuries are also present. Enhanced activity also has less direct consequences for the overall environment (land use and overuse).

Exercise Testing

At one point, American medical organizations were advocating a full clinical examination for any adult over the age of 30 years who wished to become physically active. They further recommended that the resting electrocardiogram should be supplemented by a stress electrocardiogram in subjects over 35 years old (Cooper, 1970), at a cost of $150-$200 per individual.

If 10 million adults should suddenly decide to become physically active, such a policy would create a $2 billion start-up cost for any government or private medical insurance scheme. Fortunately, this danger has been appreciated (Orban, 1974). Moreover, it has been argued that a normal and ostensibly healthy adult faces little risk from a gradual progression of physical activity if he or she first completes a simple self-administered screening tool (the PAR-Q questionnaire, Chisholm et al., 1975). Little evidence exists to show that the alternative of an expensive laboratory stress test offers more certain protection against an exercise-induced catastrophe (Shephard, 1982a; 1983a). A three-tiered test strategy of self-administered paramedical and clinical stress tests has thus been proposed (Orban, 1974).

Self-Administered Tests. At the simplest level is a self-administered fitness test. This serves as a motivational tool and provides a rough guide to an appropriate exercise prescription. The need is currently well met by the Canadian Home Fitness Kit (Shephard, 1979). The cost (current retail price of about $10) is not high enough to be a significant barrier to exercise participation, and the cost is normally borne by the individual family. Test marketing of the Fitness Kit suggested one major problem—a substantial number of families lacked a functional record player, and were thus unable to conduct the test. Results from the same marketing survey suggested that the package was favorably received by those with the necessary playback equipment. However, a need remains for a more formal evaluation of (a) the immediate and long-term motivational impact of the kit and (b) the appropriateness of the self-prescribed exercise.

Paramedical Testing. Paramedical testing is at a second level of sophistication. Commercial charges for this type of service vary quite widely, and some organizations undoubtedly have not costed their test procedures very precisely. One recent analysis put the current economic price at a minimum of $10.44 per test (Shephard, 1981; 1984). This figure depends somewhat upon location (office costs vary from $80 per m² per year for a relatively spartan suburban facility to $200 per m² per year in a well-appointed downtown development). A more significant variable is the coefficient of utilization. Very careful scheduling is necessary to test at a reasonable laboratory capacity of 4000 people per year, and many well organized stress testing units evaluate no more than 1000-1200 subjects per annum. Moreover, the $10.44 cost estimate makes no allowance for the cost of training staff, medical cover, evaluation of electrocardiograms, or the profit of an entrepreneur.

A fleet of fitness vans sponsored by the Province of Ontario offer one example of market costs. Operators were able to maintain a mobile fitness laboratory, pay staff, and offer a comprehensive fitness test with exercise prescription for a sum of $15-30 per participant while traveling widely across the province.

An even more striking example of what can be achieved by effective scheduling is provided by the Home Fitness Test trials in Saskatoon (Bailey et al., 1974; Bailey, Shephard, & Mirwald, 1976). Age- and sex-matched groups of 16 subjects performed either a cycle ergometer test or a step test under the immediate supervision of a physician, a coronary care nurse, and a team of physical education specialists. The test lasted no more than 10 min, heart rates were counted accurately by cardiotachometer, and all abnormal ECG records were printed out immediately for study by the supervising physician. The cost per test was estimated at the equivalent of $6.31 in current dollars (Shephard, 1981; 1984). This figure included hourly salaries for all personnel including the physician, plus the actual expenses of equipment leasing. In a commercial operation an additional allowance would be needed for use of 100 m³ of space (costing $3000 per month, serviced; capacity about 12,000 tests per month, costing $0.25 per test). Given efficient utilization, a physician-supervised test thus need cost no more than $6.56 per patient; however, relatively few cities could permanently sustain such a test volume, except with recourse to a mobile facility.

Clinical Stress Testing. Clinical stress testing is best reserved for a high-risk group of individuals, identified by a combination of adverse responses to self-administered questionnaires, an unsatisfactory outcome of a self-administered or paramedical exercise test, and simple clinical questioning by a health professional. The likelihood of obtaining correct and useful diagnostic or prognostic information is much enhanced if the test procedure is restricted to a population with a high risk of disease (Shephard, 1982a; 1983a). The usual costs of an annual medical examination, followed by an exercise test performed in a clinical laboratory, are substantially lower in Canada than in the U.S. Possible items to include in the account for such services are shown in Table 6.1; note that even in Canada some physicians bill their patients for larger amounts than the standard charges noted in this schedule.

Value of Testing. Repeating exercise tests at least annually on healthy adults is common, whereas patients involved in clinical rehabilitation programs are reevaluated several times per year. Testing could thus become a substantial item in any cost/benefit analysis. The practical value of much of our present exercise testing needs critical scrutiny (Shephard, 1982a,

Table 6.1 Schedule of Benefits Provided Under Ontario Hospital Insurance Plan

Test	Cost
Annual health examination	$ 27.60
Maximal stress ECG	
Technical component	23.40
Professional component	35.40
Vital capacity, $FEV_{1.0}$	
Technical component	9.20
Professional component	4.60
Total	$100.20

Note. From January 1, 1983 Ontario Hospital Insurance plan from the Ontario Ministry of Health.

No scale of charges is yet established for determinations of body fat or muscle strength.

1983a). While there can be little objection if an individual continues a program of self-evaluation, little evidence exists to show that more expensive tests are effective either in identifying individuals for whom exercise is hazardous or in prescribing a safe intensity of exercise. The best that can be obtained from such procedures is a very rough recommendation. Personal monitoring is necessary to ensure that appropriate adjustments are made for (a) interindividual variations in the energy cost of various types of exercise, (b) seasonal changes in climate, and (c) other environmental variables.

Industrial Exercise Facilities

The costs of an exercise facility vary enormously with its location and its luxury, but a few simple calculations will indicate the order of expense that may be incurred. The usual criterion for evaluation is the cost per participant-year, or (if operation is on an intermittent or seasonal basis) the cost per user-hour (Webster & Reich, 1976). However, for some purposes adding allowances for user satisfaction and complementarity with other programs is useful.

Practicality of Industrial Exercise Programs. Many authors have commended the work site as the most cost-effective location for exercise programing (Brennan, 1982a, b; Novelli & Ziska, 1982; Ware, 1982; Karson, 1982; Beck, 1982; Merwin & Northrop, 1982; Roccella, 1982). In addition to the obvious savings in time and transportation costs, avenues of program promotion are largely established, attendance is on a regular basis, colleagues provide positive reinforcement of lifestyle change, and (if blue-collar industries are selected) target groups are addressed.

Few disagree that a large corporation provides an effective vehicle for program delivery, but unfortunately surprisingly few people are employed by large companies. One U.S. survey showed that 68% of employees were in companies with fewer than 250 employees, 54% were in settings of 100 workers or less, and 42% were in establishments with a payroll of less than 50 individuals (U.S. Dept. of Commerce, 1977). In Ontario, the figures are fairly similar (55.3% in units employing fewer than 200 workers, 48.2% in groups of fewer than 100 workers, and 41.8% in companies with fewer than 50 workers; Berger, 1983). In France (Coronio & Muret, 1973), 78.5% of the companies employ less than 200 people. Possible alternatives for small organizations are noted in Table 6.2. Gray, Young, and Ennis (1983) argued that in small companies the most effective tactic for the promotion of increased physical activity might be the simple provision of shower and changing facilities. Costs per

Table 6.2 Costs of Providing Shower and Changing Facilities

Location	Cost of Facility ($)	Cost Per Worker ($)
Medium-sized factory (200 workers per shift)	4,410	22
Small factory (10 men, 2 women)	2,719	227
Small office (3 men, 1 woman)	2,058	515

Note. Based on data of J.A.M. Gray, A. Young, and J.R. Ennis, 1983. Promotion of exercise at work, *British Medical Journal, 286*, 1958-1959.
Costs expressed in 1983 Canadian dollars.

worker would range from $22 for 200 employees to $227 for 10 men and 2 women. In the U.K. it was suggested that this capital investment could be at least partially offset by reducing the rather generous statutory requirement for lavatories. Moreover, under the 1971 Finance Act, the British government allows deduction of capital costs from corporate profits on the basis that any type of exercise facility is provided for the welfare of the workers.

Scale of Facilities. The recommended floor area for an in-house industrial exercise facility ranges from 0.25 m² to 1.20 m² of floor space per employee, with a minimum floor area of 150 m² (Collis, 1977; Campbell, 1979). At the low end of this scale, a 150 m² room would meet the needs of a company employing 600 workers. Assuming also a normal class participation rate of 20% and providing for a maximum of 33% participation, 10 sets of classes per week could accommodate the needs of 200 exercisers. Allowing each class member three 50-min sessions per week plus a 10-min interclass interval, the exercise area would need to function at about 75% efficiency (30 hrs per week) to satisfy employee demands. The practicality of such heavy scheduling depends on company policy. Given a "flex time" arrangement, the 30 hrs could be accumulated by 2 hrs of operation before beginning work, 2 hrs at lunchtime, and 2 hrs after work. If a company had a shift-work system, it would be even easier to accommodate all interested employees over a 24-hr day.

In an optimum facility, the base allowance of space would be supplemented by a further 50 m² for subjects who wish to exercise on their own, plus 30 m² of office space for the fitness director and secretary. Putting the cost of such serviced space at $30 per m² per month, the total

Table 6.3 Cost of Alternative Tactics for Delivery of Employee Fitness Programs for Companies of Varying Size

Expected Number of Participants	Recommended Facility	Cost Per Participant-Year
< 400	Campus-wide facility with full-time supervisor	$300-500
5-50	Minimal facility, testing and exercise prescription only (? visiting team)	$150-500
75-250	150-300 m² facility with part- or full-time supervisor	$365-500
400-850	600-1,200 m² facility* with full-time supervisor	$300-500

*If participation rate is 20%, 600 m² for 400 participants provides a space standard of 0.3 m² per worker.

Note. Based in part on a concept of R.S. Wanzel, 1979, "Rationale for Employee Fitness Programs." In: *Employee Fitness, the How To.* Ed: R.S. Wanzel (pp. 1-16), Toronto: Ontario Ministry of Culture and Recreation.

All costs now expressed in 1983 dollars.

space cost per year would become 230 × 30 × 12, or $82,800 ($138 per worker-year, but $690 per participant-year). Some U.S. companies include sums of this order in the operating budgets of their fitness facilities, although it often remains possible either to discover basement space that is unused or to develop a cheap alternative such as a roof-top "bubble." The salaries of the fitness coordinator and secretary (with fringe benefits), any construction costs (particularly if "unused" space is to be adapted), equipment costs, and a towel service (if this is to be provided) must be added to the costs of space rental and occupancy. Using "free" space, the current cost of an employee fitness program amounts to about $80 per employee per year, or (with 20% participation) $400 per participant-year (Table 6.3). If occupancy of high-quality dedicated space is assumed, the construction item should be replaced by a rental charge; this method of calculation increases the cost to about $150 per employee per year, or $750 per participant per year.

Groups such as YMCAs are sometimes able to offer classes at lower annual fees than might be anticipated from the foregoing discussion. This reflects a combination of (a) voluntary donations toward capital costs, (b) arrangement of classes with more than 20 nominal participants, (c) space utilization exceeding 30 hrs per week, and (d) choice of a midtown or suburban rather than a prime downtown location.

Future Planning. With regard to the future, Collis (1977) has argued that fitness facilities should be included when planning any new factory or office. He maintains that architects are currently allowed up to 1% of project costs for purely aesthetic features, and that in a similar fashion about 3% of capital outlay should be invested in a fitness/life-style center. Assuming that the average office worker occupies a total of 20 m² of working and communal space (including rest rooms, cafeteria, and corridors), the proposed allowance (3% of 20 m² = 0.6 m²) would substantially exceed the previous minimum recommendation of 0.25 m² of gymnasium space per worker.

Equipment Needs. Equipment such as tape decks, record turntables, amplifiers, and loud-speakers has substantial commercial value. Thus provision must be made for securing and insuring such items. Some gymnasia make extensive investments in weight-training apparatus, but this is not a cost-effective tactic, particularly in an office where the majority of employees are female (Peepre, 1978; Marsden, 1979). Relatively few women are interested in vigorous muscle building, and even among men health benefits are probably greater if most of the available exercise time is allocated to cardiovascular training.

Maintenance. The fitness area must be kept scrupulously clean, and the operating budget or leasing contract should reflect an appropriate allowance for both normal janitorial service and a regular, thorough cleaning of floors and showers. This need can be satisfied within the basic rental charge if serviced space is costed at $30 per m² per month.

Accident Insurance. In most jurisdictions, claims arising from accidents in the employee fitness facility would be covered by a Workmen's Compensation scheme. Given a well-run program, the injury experience should not increase compensation costs—indeed, some types of manual work premiums might be reduced because of a smaller incidence of industrial injuries (chapter 4).

Public Recreational Facilities

Public recreational facilities are generally less cost-efficient than company fitness programs. Often a substantial opportunity cost is involved in travel to the facility. Usage also tends to be concentrated on weekends, and further expenditures are incurred for transportation (vehicle mileage, road systems) and parking cars. Recent patterns of governmental expenditures are summarized in Tables 6.4 and 6.5.

Public Parks. Public parks fall into three broad categories—municipal parks and parkettes, regional parks, and provincial or national parks.

Table 6.4 Governmental Expenditures on Recreational Facilities*

Level of Expenditure	1970	1972	1974	1976	1977
Federal	141M	115M	141M	216M	178M
Provincial and municipal	864M	1,199M	1,879M	2,062M	2,221M
Total (% of GNP)	—	0.43	0.57	—	—

*This total includes all facilities serving predominantly recreational ends such as stadiums, community centers, swimming pools, beaches, marinas, golf courses, skating rinks, amusement parks, exhibition facilities, parks, and playgrounds.

By way of comparison, the United Kingdom government's expenditures on parks and sport centers increased from the equivalent of $609M in 1970 to $2,184M in 1980 (Butson, 1983). The British figures include expenditures on the preservation of historic buildings and monuments and combines capital and operating costs.

Note. Based on data from *Travel, Tourism and Outdoor Recreation—A Statistical Digest 1978 and 1979* by Statistics Canada, 1981, Ottawa: Statistics Canada.

Expressed in 1983 Canadian dollars.

Table 6.5 Distribution of Canadian Governmental Expenditures on Recreational Facilities

Item	Annual Average							
	1964-66		1967-69		1970-72		1973-75	
	($)	(%)	($)	(%)	($)	(%)	($)	(%)
Theaters, arenas, amusement and recreational buildings	3.87B	83.6	3.19B	77.6	3.39B	69.2	7.23B	76.8
Park systems	638M	13.8	787M	19.1	1.093B	22.3	1.626B	17.2
Swimming pools, tennis courts, and outdoor recreational facilities	122M	2.6	136M	3.3	421M	8.5	564M	6.0
Total	4.63B		4.12B		4.90B		9.42B	

Note. From Statistics Canada, 1979b.

Municipal Parks and Parkettes. Municipal parks are, with few exceptions, little used. Gold (1972) estimated that in the U.S. they were occupied by only 5% of a community at any given time, and peak use seldom exceeded 20% of the population served. Personal observation of municipal parks around the world suggests a low occupancy of most smaller local parks and open spaces. Lick (1975) presented more optimistic data from San Jose, CA; 67% of adult individuals within a quarter of a mile radius claimed to use the park facilities that were under survey.

Factors blamed for poor usage coefficients in the U.S. included (a) an apparent desire for fantasy rather than self-oriented recreation, (b) prohibition of social pleasures such as drinking and dancing in parks, (c) poor topography and landscaping, (d) emphasis on organized programs rather than spontaneity, (e) physical dangers from the deviant behavior of other users, and (f) in poorer areas, travel distance (Kraus, 1971). To this list may be added poor planning, in particular a failure to consider client needs when deciding upon the type and scale of park that should be developed (Murphy, Williams, Niepoth, & Brown, 1973; Parker, 1971).

Regional, Provincial, and National Parks. Middle- and upper-class families use regional conservation-type parks more extensively than local parkettes. A detailed budget for a regional park is presented in Table 6.6. Opportunities are provided for swimming (changing area, sandy beach with lifeguards), outdoor informal games (a flat field), short walks (nature trail), picnics (tables, barbecues, and refreshment stand), camping, and cross-country skiing in winter. The land for this particular park was purchased at a relatively low cost about 22 years ago as part of a flood-control project. At capacity (5000 users), the direct cost is about $108 per user-year; users meet about 21.7% of the overall expenses through admission fees. From a formal economic point of view, the overall cost to society is overstated because no allowance has been made for the benefits of flood control, increases in neighboring property values, or the stimulation of local commerce. Nor is it clearly established that admission revenues have been maximized. One survey of a U.S. state park (Clawson & Knetsch, 1966) found that some users would be willing to pay the current equivalent of $14.80-18.50 for admission to the facility. At this period, user charges were meeting about 15% of park and recreational expenditures in cities such as Los Angeles (Kavanagh, Marcus, & Gay, 1973). In Ontario, an average of 27% of operating costs for sports and recreational programs is currently derived from fees and service charges. For a regional park (Table 6.6), revenues ($3.00 per car admitted) met 21.7% of total costs but 55.8% of operating costs.

At present, the most useful parkland pursuits for maintaining health seem to be swimming and cross-country skiing. Unfortunately, a serious limitation of many parks is that the seasons for such activities are short. In the example of Table 6.6, the park effectively operates at capacity (1100 car admissions at $3 each) for no more than 45 days per year. An alternative possibility for parkland development is to build fitness trails of the Parcourse type, at a cost of about $8000 for a 3 km circuit (Thomas, 1979).

Table 6.6 Cost Data for a Metropolitan Toronto Conservation Authority Park With an Area of 275 Acres (110 Hectares) and a Capacity of About 5,000 People and Parking for 1,100 Cars*

Park Costs		Annual Cost
Land acquisition costs (275 acres) $645,000†		
Investment at 15%		$ 96,750
Development costs		
(a) Changing room and refreshment booth	$ 250,000	
(b) Dam	200,000	
(c) Workshop	150,000	
(d) Roads (3.2 km) and parking	400,000	
(e) Landscaping (grass, trees, nature trails, ski trails, maple syrup demonstration)	150,000	
(f) Picnic tables (650) and barbecues	100,000	
(g) Tools (mowers, shovels, ski equipment)	100,000	
(h) Vehicles (trucks, tractors, snowblowers)	75,000	
Total	$1,425,000	
Capital investment at 15%		213,750
Depreciation of (a), (b), (c), (d), and (e) at 5%		57,500
Depreciation of (f), (g), and (h) at 20%		55,000
Operating costs		
Materials (including taxes, utilities, insurance)		105,800
Labor (5 full-time park employees, 5 lifeguards, 2 gate keepers, 1 extra		163,000
Total per year		$691,800

Revenue = $150,000 per year. Cost per user-year = $108.36.

*Expressed in 1983 Canadian dollars.

†Because of expressway construction and metropolitan growth, costs at this particular site would currently exceed $2,345 per acre.

Note. Courtesy of Mr. Jim Agnew, Metropolitan Toronto Conservation Authority.

Indoor Facilities. Typical costs of some sport facilities are summarized in Tables 6.7 and 6.8. The expense per taxpayer depends on the participation rate (a figure of 20% has been assumed, although this may be high for a community-based operation) and the efficiency of scheduling facility use. Land is generally a major cost. The current price varies widely from urban and suburban to small-town locations, and costs could possibly be greatly reduced if speculation in building land were curbed. Moreover, much land is purchased for parking space rather than for the facility itself; this aspect of cost could be reduced if public transportation were improved or if a network of centers were established within walking or cycling distance of every home.

Table 6.7 Operating Costs for a Gymnasium

Operating Costs		$ (Million)
(a) Land costs* (4 acres) $0.8 million		
Investment at 15%		$0.12
(b) Construction		
Building—1,000 m² at $600/m²	$0.60 million	
Parking	$0.20 million	
Investment at 15%		0.12
Depreciation at 5%		0.04
(c) Salaries		0.048
(d) Equipment—$20,000		
(Investment at 15%, depreciation at 20%)		0.007
(e) Specific maintenance		0.010
(f) Supplies (including heat, telephone, and utilities)		0.020
Total		$0.365

*Land costs vary widely, depending on location.

Note. A floor area of 1,000 m² provides space for 1,000/7.5, or up to 133 participants at any given time. With 10 groups of users, the cost at capacity is $274 per user-year.

Based in part on data provided by Ontario Ministry of Tourism and Recreation.

The annual costs of operating a hockey arena or a 25 m pool are relatively similar, while a gymnasium is somewhat cheaper, mainly because of lower construction costs.

Some budgets show 1/3-1/2 of the operating cost being met from potential revenues (admissions, membership fees, club rentals, instructional fees, pro shops, and concessions). However, this is not necessarily a desirable trend in a public facility—user fees may deter target groups such as the unemployed, low-paid workers, and the elderly, while periodic rental of the entire facility to specialist clubs leads to an erratic admission schedule, discouraging general public attendance.

The cost per participant depends on the time for which each person is allowed to use any given type of facility and the floor density that is accepted. The maximum recommended occupancy of a 25 m pool is about 100 swimmers, but people will be unlikely to stay in the water more than 30 min. A capacity of at least 2000 people per pool per day can thus be assumed (cost: $60 per citizen-year).

An ice-hockey game may involve 2 teams of 25 players each for up to 2 hrs of ice time. A typical day might allow the scheduling of 4 games, providing physical activity for 200 people. This suggests the high cost

Table 6.8 Summary of Operating Costs for Various Types of Recreational Facilities, Assuming All Potential Participants Seek Use on a Given Day, With 20% Community Participation

Facility	Cost Per Participant-Year	Cost Per Citizen
Conservation area	$ 108	$ 20.40
Tennis*	946	189.20
Soccer field		
With spectators	4,528	905.60
Without spectators	1,807	361.40
Gymnasium	274	54.80
Ice arena (indoor)		
Hockey	2,665	533.00
Public skating	178^x	35.60
Swimming pool (indoor)	300†	60.00

*Tennis would be more expensive if it was not neighborhood based; neither parking nor administrative supervision has been assumed necessary.

^{x}Public skating is calculated for a very heavy ice-density. All of the figures cited depend on maximized occupancy.

†Swimming has been calculated on a relatively short water time (30 min or less).

of $2665 per player per year. However, with 20% community participation, the annual cost would drop to $533 per community resident. It may also be unfair to assume that the average player will engage in a 2-hr game more than 2 or 3 times per week, while many municipalities allow only 1, rather than 2, hours of ice time for most teams; with efficient scheduling, costs could thus drop to $190 per resident-year, or less. Public skating can be even more economical. Assuming that a 3-hr public session allows access by 1000 people and that three such sessions can be scheduled at capacity per day, the cost is only $35.60 per citizen per year.

Gymnasia can be built for about $600/m². The minimum floor space per participant is about 7.5 m², depending on the type of gymnastics to be undertaken, so that the capacity of a 1000-m² hall is about 133 people. Effective training can be accomplished with 40-50 min floor sessions, so that a capacity of at least 1330 users per day can be assumed (cost: $54.80 per citizen-year). The cost of British sports centers is of a similar order (Table 6.9).

Mixed-Use Facilities. Schemes can be envisaged in which the costs of gymnastics and sports centers are subsidized by mixed land arrangements

Table 6.9 Cost of Indoor Sport Halls in the United Kingdom*

Facility	Cost Per Unit	Planned Provision
Sport halls		
Large district	$5.70M	341
Small district	1.80M	134
Small rural or urban	0.58M	682
Converted buildings	0.50M	470
Adapted buildings	0.066M	1,507

*Expressed in 1983 Canadian dollars.

Note. From *A Forward Look* (p. 13) by U.K. Sports Council, 1982, London: Author.

Table 6.10 An Example of Commercial Financing of a Sport Center Proposed for the U.K.*

Items	Expense	Income
Construction estimate	$470,000	
(Fees, finance, contingencies, delay costs)		
Rental to local municipality	$250,000	
(Capitalized at 10%)		
Shortfall	$220,000	
Petrol service station		$100,000
(Rental capitalized at 10%)		
Offices	$481,000	
(Rental of 740 m² at $65 per m²)		
Construction costs	$361,000	$120,000
	$220,000	$220,000

*Shortfall of costs met by income from offices and a service station.

Note. From "Raising Finance for Recreation Facilities" by R. Bidgood, 1972, *Parks and Sports Grounds,* **38,** pp. 141-144.

(Table 6.10). Thus Bidgood (1972) has illustrated how 40-50% of the costs of an indoor sports center could be countered by revenues from adjacent offices and a service station. In this context, Jenkins, in Roberts (1979) offers an interesting comment on the commercial provision of leisure facilities: "The wicked face of capitalism is true only if it takes advantage of its monopoly position, a position which the local authority can redress through its control of planning permission" (p. 23).

Table 6.11 Amount of Sponsorship Support Given to Particular Sports in the U.K.

Sport	Support
Motor racing	$13,800T
Horse racing	3,220T
Golf	2,300T
Association football	1,380T
Cricket	1,240T
Lawn tennis	1,060T
Equestrianism	920T
Cycling	920T
Olympics	506T
Sailing	460T
Athletics	440T

Note. From *Commercial Sponsorship of Sport and Other Activities in the U.K.* by System Three (Communications) Ltd., 1973, London: System Three Communications, cited in *The Financing of Sport in the United Kingdom* (p. 41) by the U.K. Sports Council, 1983.

All values for support here expressed in 1983 Canadian dollars.

Table 6.12 Ranking of Sport Sponsorship by Industry

Rank	Industry	Percent of Total Support
1	Tobacco	40.7
2	Oil	18.3
3	Tires	10.0
4	Brewing	7.6
5	Finance	4.2
6	Food	3.4
7	Retail clothing and sports goods	3.4
8	Wines and spirits	3.3
9	Bookmakers	2.9
10	Other	6.2

Note. From *Commercial Sponsorship of Sport and Other Activities in the U.K.* by System Three (Communications) Ltd., 1973, London: System Three Communications, cited in *The Financing of Sport in the United Kingdom* (p. 41) by the U.K. Sports Council, 1983.

Sponsorship Arrangements. A second commercial source of funding is sponsorship (Table 6.11). Unfortunately, the potential sponsors are often companies that market products with an adverse effect upon health (Table 6.12), and much of the support is directed to commercial spectator sport. A recent study (Council of Executive Directors, 1983) suggested that

Canadian corporate sponsors contributed about $50M per year to various types of fitness, recreation, and amateur sport programs (about $6.25 per worker-year). John Hudson, current Director of Media Properties for the Labatt Brewing Company, explained motivations as follows: "We put $24.5M into Canadian professional sport this year because we get financial return on our investment." However, $5.5M was donated to amateur sport "largely . . . because the competition contributes too" (p. 6). At least $10.6M of the $50M donated to amateur sport organizations came from beer, liquor, and tobacco firms, and beneficiaries included rugger, soccer, tennis, curling, skiing, golf, bowling, equestrian, and auto sport groups.

Public- Versus Private-Sector Involvement. The relative contribution of public and private sectors to the provision of leisure facilities has been discussed in chapter 3. In North America, the four main activities that are pursued at commercial facilities are squash, dancing, golf, and curling. Most other vigorous pursuits are either followed at public and nonprofit installations, or take place out of doors without any special facilities. Ritchie, in Roberts (1979, p. 14), concluded that "based on past experience, it (would be) optimistic to expect major recreational facilities to be sponsored by the private sector" in Canada.

Outdoor Pursuits. Costs can be reduced by playing outdoor sports because the construction of buildings accounts for 40-50% of the expense of an indoor program (Table 6.8). The penalty of an outdoor emphasis is often a very short operating season—the water becomes too cold for swimming or the ground gets too hard for playing soccer. Although the outdoor environment is aesthetically more pleasing than a minimum cost indoor sport center, if the season length can be doubled by providing an indoor facility, the extra expense can generally be justified.

Specific calculations are presented for tennis and soccer. The cost of outdoor tennis courts is now quite well established. The expense to a community is substantially reduced if the courts are near enough to avoid driving (no parking area), while both the playing season and the hours of daily use can be increased by providing floodlights. Finally, in many locations the day-to-day administration of the courts can be handled by a local taxpayer association. With such economies, the cost of this type of activity is about $189 per citizen-year; in many instances, use of the land is further extended by winter skating on the court surface.

Many authors recommend a site of at least 10 acres for a soccer or a football pitch; this allows for parking and the building of substantial stands for spectators. Given minimal parking and no spectator stands, the cost is still about $1807 per citizen-year. This figure would be increased if changing and shower areas were installed and if the season was extended by providing artificial turf. Data from the U.K. (Sports Council, 1982a, b) shows that providing minimal changing and ancillary accommodations at established pitches would require a capital cost of $85,000, while installing an artificial playing surface would cost $32,000 per unit.

Personal Costs

Unarguably, high personal costs are incurred with competitive involvement in most types of sport (Morikawa, 1979; Ellis, 1982). Top Japanese gymnasts each spend the equivalent of $37,000 • yr^{-1}. In Ontario, the 1% of the population who are elite performers or enthusiasts in any discipline each spend $600-4000 • yr^{-1} on participation in their chosen sports.

Luxury activities can be costly even for the less-committed individuals. Olsen (1983, March) priced downhill skiing at $3000 • yr^{-1} and tennis at $2000 or more per year. Even activities such as jogging and running carry an appreciable expense. Neglecting the probable costs of additional food ($50-300, depending on the distance run and the diet selected, chapter 2), likely expenditures on clothing, equipment, and travel range from a little over $200 per year for the "thrifty runner" to as much as $5000-6000 per year for the enthusiast who takes a spouse to distance meets (Shephard, 1981; Olsen, 1983).

Low-Cost Pursuits. The main attraction of a walking, jogging, or running program, from the viewpoint of public administration, is that both personal and governmental costs are kept to a minimum. If an indoor track is used in winter, this may require a subsidy, but indoor shopping precincts and large office complexes allow much exercise using existing space. Moreover, with appropriate adjustments in the amount of clothing worn, it remains quite feasible to continue outdoor walking throughout most U.S. and Canadian winters. Indeed, some degree of cold exposure may pay the useful bonus of encouraging fat loss (O'Hara, Allen, Shephard, & Allen, 1979).

Implications for Town Planning. Reference has already been made to the desirability of incorporating provisions for walkers and cyclists into the planning of new towns. Small design features can do much to encourage physical activity—planting shade trees for summer, grading to avoid winter icing of sidewalks, and ensuring an adequate set-back of tall buildings to minimize wind-funneling. If citizens are encouraged to incorporate walking and cycling into their normal daily routines, the various levels of government will benefit from a reduced pressure on roads and mass transportation systems. In Toronto, for example, the 30% operating subsidy of the Metropolitan Transit Commission costs over $120 million per year, about $160 per wage earner per year. Much of the loss is incurred on poorly patronized "feeder" bus routes that operate over distances that most citizens could conveniently cover on foot or by bicycle.

Medical Supervision

Some further comments may be offered on the costs and benefits of providing full medical supervision for exercise testing and prescription.

Risks of Exercise Testing. Fatalities during exercise testing occur almost exclusively in patients with known cardiovascular disease (Rochmis & Blackburn, 1971). But even in such individuals, problems are infrequent. One episode of ventricular fibrillation has been observed for every 8000 submaximal tests performed on postcoronary patients (Shephard, Kavanagh, Tuck, & Kennedy, 1983). Given the immediate proximity of equipment for cardiac resuscitation, the risk of death for such patients is about 1 in 40,000 to 1 in 50,000. Assuming also that the net worth of a postcoronary patient is $300,000 (20 years of further work at $15,000 per annum*), an appropriate insurance allowance might be $6.00-7.50 per test.

When a submaximal test is performed on an ostensibly healthy adult, the risk of an emergency is much lower than that seen in testing patients from a cardiac rehabilitation program. The hazard may be calculated on the basis that it is less than that encountered in endurance sport (Shephard, 1977a) or greater than that observed under resting conditions. The latter approach indicates a somewhat greater danger, and it is probably correct because problems due to the self-selection of athletes are then avoided. The chances of a cardiac incident (fatal or nonfatal) while resting are about 1 in 300 per year in middle-aged men and 1 in 1000 per year in middle-aged women, or (with a population of both sexes) 1 in 22.8 million every 15 min. Exercise increases the danger by a factor of at least five (giving a risk of 1 in 4.6 million over 15 min), but with 80% successful resuscitation the death rate from brief submaximum testing should be no more than 1 in 22.8 million. Again, setting patient worth at $300,000, insurance could be provided for about 1.3 cents per test.

Note. Some patients will of course have higher potential salaries. Parr and Kerr (1975) have thus recommended providing personal liability insurance to the current equivalent of $1,000,000, with additional coverage for the hospital or university providing the test facilities.

Physician Versus Paramedical Supervision. How would the presence of a physician influence this outcome? A slightly greater chance of successful cardiac resuscitation might exist, although in practice the physician is unlikely to improve upon the success rate of a well trained paramedical professional. Unfortunately, the presence of a physician also seems to increase the risk of a person developing ventricular fibrillation during a test. Part of the increment may be spurious—an expression of the fact that physicians see individuals in whom problems are likely—but much of the increase is a real phenomenon which is a reaction to the anxiety generated by recourse to a doctor. The provision of direct medical cover for a 15-min submaximum exercise test on a healthy adult is, moreover, highly cost-ineffective. Even ignoring the worsening of prognosis induced by the doctor's white coat, at $35 per test the cost would be ($35 × 4.6 million), $161 million for every emergency attended, or at least $201 million for every successful resuscitation. Plainly, a much more effective tactic is to train paramedical professionals in cardiopulmonary resuscitation. This would cost, at most, $50 per year, 1.25 cents per subject tested (assuming a capacity of 4000 tests per year), or 0.0125 × 4.6 million ($57,500) for every emergency attended.

Risks of Exercise Programs. Some risks exist in the training process itself (Koplan, Powell, Sikes, Shirley, & Campbell, 1982). Parallel calculations can thus cost the provision of various types of supervised exercise programs. Assuming a class size of 40-50 patients and allowing 1 hr of physician time, 1 hr of gym time, and 2-1/2 hrs of physical activity supervisor time per session, Pyfer and Doane (1973) calculated operating costs at the equivalent of $12.15 per person-session for the first 3 months of postcoronary rehabilitation, $10.80 per person-session for the next 9 months, and $5.40 thereafter. Zohman (1973) cited a similar cost of $13.50 per person-session of supervised cycle ergometer exercise. The Toronto Rehabilitation Centre uses 1 physician and 4 supervisors for a group of 50 cardiac patients (Shephard, 1977a); the cost is about $170 per session ($3.40 per person-session) excluding gymnasium rental. How do these costs match the risks?

One recent survey of unsupervised Rhode Island joggers (Thompson, Funk, Carleten, & Sturner, 1982) found one death per 396,000 hrs of jogging. The experience of U.S. YMCAs (one fatal or nonfatal event per 495,971 person-hours of activity, Vander, Franklin, & Rubenfire, 1982) was of the same general order. Haskell (1978) further suggested that for well-run postcoronary exercise classes, the risk was one event per 268,922 person-hours. Again, putting the value of the individual at $300,000, and assuming an 80% success rate for cardiac resuscitation, the annual cost of insurance for three 1-hour sessions of activity per week would be about

$$\frac{150 \times 300,000 \times 20}{500,000 \times 100} = \$18$$

for an ostensibly healthy individual and about twice as much for a post-coronary patient.

Supervision of Exercise Programs. Given a class size of 50 members, the risk of a cardiac incident during a 1-hour class session is about 1 in 10,000 for ostensibly healthy adults and 1 in 5000 for postcoronary patients. At $105 per hour, the cost of medical supervision is in itself about $1.05 million per incident in a supposedly healthy population, and (because incidents are more probable) $0.52 million per incident for a postcoronary class. The total cost of the Pyfer and Doane program is $1.7-3.8 million per incident, while the Toronto Rehabilitation Centre program costs $0.85 million per incident.

About 50% of high-risk individuals could be eliminated from a supposedly healthy sample by using a simple, self-administered screening questionnaire. This would have the effect of increasing the cost of medical supervision of normal adults to $2.1 million per incident. Assuming also an 80% success rate for resuscitation, the cost per success would amount to $2.63 million in "normals" and $0.65 million in postcoronary patients. Unfortunately, no guarantee exists that the presence of a physician would materially improve the proportion of successful resuscitations. Indeed, the "white coat syndrome" might actually increase the number of incidents occurring during physical activity. Thus it may be concluded that in most situations medical supervision of an exercise program is not cost-effective. As during exercise testing, a much cheaper and safer approach is to teach the techniques of cardiopulmonary resuscitation to both paramedical professionals and the general public.

Indirect Costs

There are also the indirect costs associated with attaining physical fitness.

Personal Injuries

Researchers often point out that the potential economic savings of a vigorous fitness program can be offset by the adverse effects of recreational injuries (Toplin & Bentkover, 1980; Sorensen & Sonne-Holm, 1981).

Table 6.13 Incidence of Disabling Injuries in Industrial Recreation for a Factory Employing 3,100 Workers

Type of Activity	Incidence (Per Million Person-Hours of Play or Practice)	Time Loss Per Injury (Days)
Basketball	257	14.2
Softball	249	26.1
Table tennis	234	21.0
Baseball	82	24.5
Bowling	14	2.7
Golf	0	0
Tennis	0	0
All sports	75	19.8

Cost of replacement labor = \$66 × 1.75 = \$115 per day

If 20% participation, 150 hrs activity per year, work loss = $\frac{75 \times 19.8 \times 150}{5 \times 1,000,000}$ =
0.045 days per worker-year = \$5.12 cost per worker-year*

Cost of injury

Medical consultation, radiographs, plaster cast \$100-200, depending on injury. Chance of injury 2.27×10^{-3}. This effective cost is \$0.23-0.45 per worker-year.†

---

*This cost has already been noted in chapter 4, which considered the net effect of physical activity upon absenteeism.

†This cost has already been noted in chapter 2, which considered the net effect of physical activity upon health care costs.

Note. From "Occupation" by J.S. Felton, 1971, In L.A. Larson (Ed.), *Encyclopedia of Sports Sciences and Medicine* (p. 968), New York: MacMillan.

Level of Risk. Data from an industrial recreational program (Felton, 1971) provide some indication of the likely magnitude of this expense (Table 6.13). On the assumption that participants engage in their chosen activities during 150 hrs of each year, a 20% program participation rate yields an average time loss of 0.045 days per worker-year. Given also a 1.75-fold replacement cost for the injured employee (\$66 per day), the expense becomes \$5.12 per worker-year. Sorensen and Sonne-Holm (1981) found that more than half of injured Danish athletes reported to work the next day, and the average time-loss was 8 days per injury.

Treatment Costs. The cost of treating a sport-related injury—typically damage to an arm or a leg—is more variable. In the Danish study, the cost of an orthopedic hospital bed was \$135 • day^{-1}, while an outpatient visit cost \$54.25 (exclusive of any special transportation). The total social cost was $467 per injury, with about two thirds of this figure attributable to lost work. Personal costs of $65 (mainly lost earnings) were also incurred. In Canada, current fee schedules suggest that the cost for outpatient treatment of a fracture might be $100-400. The average chance of incurring an injury is 2.27×10^{-3} per year. The cost of treatment is thus in the range $0.23-0.90 per worker-year; as in Denmark, the main social cost is lost work.

Details of costs depend upon the type of sport, the definition of an injury, and the vigor of competition. In intercollegiate sports the risk is apparently 10-200 times greater than in more modest competitions (Thorndike, 1942; MacIntosh, Skrien, & Shephard, 1972). Overenthusiastic participation of the employee in any sport can push the injury rate to a level that introduces a significant cost burden.

Sports Medicine Clinics. In recent years, many hospitals have opened sports medicine clinics that offer advice on the minor discomforts associated with regular exercise. Many of the conditions thus treated would previously have been dealt with informally by the participants and their friends. Careful costing of sports medicine operations is needed. In particular, a critical assessment should be made as to whether the availability of a sports medicine clinic increases or reduces the ultimate demand for orthopedic services by active individuals.

Promotional Costs

The private sector of the North American economy currently invests almost $100B per year in advertising. It thus seems logical that health education departments should benefit from this experience; they should employ a new breed of specialists with expertise in advertising, marketing, and even propaganda (Cappon, 1983, March/April).

Potential Impact of Promotional Programs. Many of those currently attracted by fitness promotions have previously been active (Santa Barbara, 1982a, b), and assessing either the impact or the cost-effectiveness of the measures that are taken to promote personal fitness is difficult (Green, 1979; Rogers et al., 1981; Godin & Shephard, 1983). One example of the potential for changing population behavior within a totalitarian regime is the "Strength through Joy" movement in the Third Reich. Through vigorous propaganda, the number of Germans participating in day-long hikes increased from 0.1 to 1.0 million between 1934 and 1936, while total participation in the movement grew from 2.3 to 8.6 million people (Spode,

1980). Maccoby and Farquhar (1975) concluded from a more recent study in southern California that, given enough time, use of the mass media to improve lifestyle was much cheaper than personal counseling, yet just as effective. There seems to be both a threshold level of exposure (below which media campaigns are a waste of money, Thornton, 1974), and a saturation level (which has certainly not yet been reached in the case of fitness promotion). Given additional exposure, television quite likely could reach current target groups (Flay & Schlegel, 1980; Olson & Zanna, 1981).

Current Expenditures. The U.S. President's Council on Fitness has quite a small budget (e.g., in 1976 the current equivalent of $1.15M; Thomas, 1979). Promotional expenditures in the U.K. total $1.86M per year (U.K. Sports Council, 1982b). Canadian data can be drawn from operations of the Crown Corporation ParticipACTION, incorporated as a nonprofit company in 1971. Over the 12 years since its foundation, the federal government has contributed a cumulative amount of $6.3 million to the ParticipACTION budget. "Hard cash" contributions from the private sector have totaled $5 million, while air and print space (100% donated) has had a normal value slightly in excess of $100 million; government has thus seen a return of about 16:1 on its advertising dollars. Among regular supporters of ParticipACTION are 145 television and cable outlets, 305 radio stations, 35 major national magazines, 200 special interest publications, and more than 500 weekly newspapers. In Canada, some additional promotion exists at the federal and provincial levels (Lawler/ Dean Partnership, 1982). In Ontario, the direct promotional budget is currently about $0.3M • yr^{-1} (6.9 cents per worker-year), with a total budget of $1.27M • yr^{-1} (29 cents per worker-year) for Fitness Ontario.

Impact of Fitness Promotion. Statistics Canada estimated that in 1971 less than 5% of the adult population was regularly active two or three times per week, compared with a current 37% of the adult population. The extent to which government-sponsored fitness promotion has contributed to this increase of physical activity is uncertain, but the change of exercise habits has been largest in the medium-sized cities of western Canada, where ParticipACTION is best known. By 1980, 85% of adult Canadians knew what ParticipACTION was, and were able to describe its functions, and in 1982, 71% of the population was able to recognize the organization from its symbol alone. Such popular awareness is probably exceeded only by McDonald's restaurants (Howell & Howell, 1982). Recognition of ParticipACTION was particularly high among the younger and more active segment of the population. Of those who had heard of ParticipACTION, 85% thought it was effective in the sense that it had caused people to become physically more active. Most advertisers would regard this as a high success rate. Thus it might be concluded that a "geared" governmental investment of less than 6 cents per worker-year had achieved a substantial penetration of the fitness market. But a discouraging fact is that many who are well-aware of programs remain inactive (A.R.A., 1981); more needs to be done to bridge the gap between awareness and activity. Older people and blue-collar workers are beginning to show interest in exercise. Nevertheless, further research is necessary to establish what changes in the amount and type of advertising expenditures would be necessary to reach the majority of these target groups.

Research

Canada is often thought to invest more in fitness research than the U.S. However, current funding is only about 5 cents per worker-year. Although this item would normally appear in a cost/benefit analysis, the sum is currently so small that it may be neglected.

The same criticism of research priorities can be leveled with other nations. In Britain, for example, the funding of fitness and sport studies has risen somewhat in recent years, but the total budget for 1983/84 included no more than $1.74M for a combination of research and information dissemination. Unfortunately, almost a quarter of this total is consumed by administrative fees.

Environmental Costs

The provision of facilities for active leisure can have a substantial impact upon urban, peri-urban, and rural environments, whether the demand be for indoor or outdoor pursuits. To quote one recent example, the opening of additional entertainment facilities at a Disneyland-type operation near Toronto created an 8 km traffic jam on all four northbound lanes of a major expressway for the first 2 hrs of a fine weekend in June 1983. In Britain, broadly defined leisure activities now account for 43% of motor vehicle use (Roberts, 1979), and in North America the percentage of leisure-related driving is probably even higher, so that the recreational use of the automobile becomes a major environmental concern.

Urban Environment.   Within the city, a hastily constructed sport hall or skating rink with poorly landscaped parking can add appreciably to suburban blight. Urban parks have been a particular political concern in some

U.S. cities, and it has been alleged that substantial charges accrue to local residents from vandalism and the need for additional policing of neighboring streets (Kavanagh et al., 1973). On the other hand, well-designed and attractively landscaped facilities not only make physical activity appealing, but also have a positive impact upon the total community environment.

Parkland and Property Values. While small property owners often oppose the development of parkland, in fact parks and conservation areas commonly augment their property values. A 65-acre extension of Central Park in New York induced a six-fold escalation of local land prices over 6 years (Jensen, 1977).

The same phenomenon has been seen elsewhere. Schutjer and Hallberg (1968) noted a downward price differential of $490 per acre on moving 1.6 km away from a regional park. Rickey (1972) reported a 3000% increase of land values following approval of a seasonal home subdivision. A detailed analysis of data for the Pearl River Reservoir development (Jackson, MI) found a 258% escalation of real estate values over the first 5 years following announcement of the project, compared with an increase of less than 50% for other nearby land (U.S. Bureau of Outdoor Recreation, 1972).

Some politicians argue that private investors should not harvest such windfall profits from public investment; the politicians suggest that compulsory land purchases should be made around parks and that further park development should be financed from profits on the resale of surplus land. (This principle is commonly applied to private developments in which prestige lots are sold to finance a golf course or a country club.) If a 640-acre tract of land is to be developed, the "gift" to the municipality of a 10-acre developed park can be more than recouped from increased property values. Local governments need to look more closely at development-density bonuses offered in return for the donation of parkland—the donation, although socially useful, may really be an investment on the part of the entrepreneur.

Other sources of income from parkland (U.S. Dept. of Commerce, 1964; Smith, Portain, & Champlin, 1966) include fishing rights (up to $7 per user-day), hunting (up to $11 per user-day), and camping (up to $7.50 per site).

Planning Recommendations

There are different kinds of planning consideration in terms of indoor and outdoor facilities.

Indoor Pursuits

Many North American municipalities provide facilities for ice hockey, figure skating, roller skating (summer use of rinks), and swimming. Gymnasia, indoor tracks, and courts for racquet sports have, to date, been operated mainly by volunteer or commercial organizations. However, now an increasing trend exists to develop municipal fitness programs, judo clubs, and the like either in purpose-built sport centers or in existing school facilities. The latter approach minimizes both financial costs and environmental impact. A suburban arena with parking can easily occupy 3-4 acres (1.2-1.6 hectares) of good agricultural land. If a single facility is large enough to accommodate the needs of 10,000 to 12,000 people, the total cost to satisfy the entire North American population would be about 350 km^2 (27,000-35,000 hectares) of prime serviced land, dropping to 70 km^2 (5200-7000 hectares) if the participation rate was 20%.

Dumazedier and Imbert (1964) set the needs of a French city of 50,000 people at 19 hectares of stadia and training space, 10 hectares of suburban parks, 12 gymnasia, 4 major swimming pools (2 covered), 1 sport hall, 3 training rooms, and 9000 m^2 of other training space.

Murphy et al. (1973) proposed rather poorer standards for the U.S.— 50,000 people served by 1 indoor pool, 5 gymnasia, 12 multi-use rooms, and 32 handball courts, supplemented by 25 tennis courts, 16 golf courses, and 32 archery ranges.

European Sport Centers.   Britain has shown great initiative in establishing its own form of indoor sport centers over the past decade. In 1970/71 only 12 sport centers existed, but by 1980/81 the provision had increased to 461 major and 310 lesser centers. A typical major facility comprises 2 large multipurpose halls, generally used for gymnastics and basketball, plus smaller rooms for such pursuits as squash, trampoline, volleyball, handball, dance, table tennis, and judo. By 1980/81, 61% of the target of one center per 40,000 to 50,000 population (Birch, 1971) had been realized. Given reasonably efficient utilization (average occupancy 60 people, 16 hrs per day), such centers would allow about 4-5% of the population to engage in a reasonable amount of physical activity. It is also planned to provide one swimming pool and 20 squash courts per 50,000 people (U.K. Sports Council, 1982a, b). The land cost of the British sport centers is, in principle, similar to that of a North American skating rink, although more dense urban housing allows a somewhat less generous provision of parking space.

In other parts of Europe, the development of sport halls is even further advanced than in Britain. For example, the Netherlands (Netherlands Sports Federation, 1980) already provide one center for every 27,000 people, which is almost twice the British standard. Meyer and Brightbill (1964) proposed a similar scale of facilities for the U.S., although they suggested that much of this need could be satisfied through the use of school buildings. They recommended providing 10 gymnasia, 25 multiple-use rooms, and 5 indoor swimming pools for a community of 100,000 people.

The Issue of Accessibility. Accessibility is vital to the effective use of both indoor and outdoor facilities. Relative to their British counterparts, North Americans would probably be prepared to invest a greater opportunity cost in traveling to a sport or fitness center. However, in the U.K., the majority of users live within 6 km of a center, a journey time of less than 15 min (Vickerman, 1975; Crompton, 1976; Arrowsmith, 1979; Atkinson & Collins, 1980; Veal, 1982). Incentives to travel farther include youth (the most mobile group are those aged 20-29 years), a substantial disposable income, involvement in competition, and the potential for reaching superior or different facilities. In Britain, convenience has apparently created demand; thus, the construction of a sport center at Atherton (Lancashire), generated 2,000 new users over 5 years, although already 7 sport centers and 12 swimming pools existed within a 10-km radius (Northwest Council for Sport and Recreation, U.K., 1982). Other newly opened centers have reported involvement of 35-50% of previously inactive people. At Torfaen (Gwent, U.K.), 83% of the population live within 3 km of the sport center, and many gain additional exercise by walking or cycling to the building. Given this favorable local environment, the participation rate at Torfaen is four times the British national average (Whaley, 1980). Little evidence shows that the new sport centers have had an adverse effect upon the use of existing voluntary and commercial facilities. If anything, a general stimulation of interest in sport and a continued use and extension of existing buildings has occurred (Jenkins, Bonser, Knapp, & Collins, 1981).

Shared-Use Facilities. Statistics from the U.K. suggest that environmental benefits are supplemented by a 40% greater direct cost-effectiveness when a facility is shared by school and community (Built Environment Research Group, 1978; Coopers & Lybrand Associates, 1981). The main objection to shared use is a negative impact upon the participation of such important target groups as housewives, shift-workers, the unemployed, and the retired. This is partly a consequence of restricted availability, and partly the negative image that some target groups find in a school environment.

Other cost-effective approaches that could improve the appearance of older urban areas include the refurbishing of large or redundant schools, used or unlet factories, and churches that are abandoned or have declining congregations. Greater use could also be made of existing hospital, university, and military facilities. A detailed inventory would reveal much unused or underused space in most cities.

Quality, Maintenance, and Public Expectations. An attractive external elevation and a pleasant internal environment do much to encourage the use of recreational space. Public expectations are continuously rising, and thus budgets should contain due provision not only to construct but also to maintain and ultimately to replace indoor sport centers. The U.K. currently faces a legacy of neglect; for example, a third of its swimming pools are antiquated buildings, predating World War I. A recent survey disclosed that more than 300 British indoor pools needed major structural work, including extensive refurbishing with replacement of water treatment and heating and ventilating systems (U.K. Sports Council, 1982a, b). In Canada, the repair budget for pools, tennis courts, and arenas is currently about 7% of annual capital investment (Ellis, 1982). Most of the existing ice rinks and pools were constructed with very little thought for energy conservation, and major redesign is becoming necessary as fuel costs rise. As much as $20,000 per year may be saved through an investment of $100,000 in an improved heating system. In some cases, updating proves to be prohibitively expensive and forces eventual conversion of a pool or rink into a dry type of sport facility. (Costs shown in Table 6.8 include a 5% depreciation allowance on all capital investments.)

Reaching Target Populations. To date, the recreational environment has been kept simple, if not austere, with a view to minimizing expense. However, it is now necessary to consider possible changes in facilities and programs that could reach target populations not currently involved in sport and fitness activities, for instance, housewives with small children, blue-collar workers, ethnic minorities, the elderly, the disabled, the unemployed, and the mentally handicapped.

Several studies have shown a disproportionate number of car owners among current participants (Arrowsmith, 1979; Atkinson & Collins, 1980; U.K. Sports Council, 1982a, b). New facilities should therefore have easy access to mass transit, place of work, or place of residence. Addition of a creche and adjustments in the timing of programs may encourage the involvement of parents with young children, while design features such as ramps, wide doorways, and modified toilets will be necessary to assure participation of the disabled. Such targeting may increase the cost of buildings by 10-25% and program operation by up to 100%, but if access is by foot or by mass transit such expenses will be at least partially offset by savings on land for parking.

Possible changes in the ambience of a recreational facility that would attract the blue-collar worker continue to be debated. Relative success is currently linked to consumer-oriented management and a wide range of price options (Whaley, 1980). It has also been argued that many blue-collar workers lack a knowledge of basic physical activity skills. Closer links are thus needed between physical educators and those designing school curricula or adult education programs. Lack of transport and admission fees are further deterrents for low-paid workers with large families, single parents, and the unemployed. Provision of better public transportation, the construction of facilities within walking distance of housing developments, and the subsidization of sport center memberships may all encourage the involvement of such individuals.

Initial recruitment is often through the persuasion of a friend, and the design of a facility must thus reflect social interaction rather than austere clinical efficiency. Possibly the commercial sector could become involved in developing the social component of sport centers. In the U.K. many sporting pursuits such as skittles, cricket, and rugger were originally linked to the village inn. Reestablishment of ties with the neighborhood pub or working men's club has thus been proposed as a means of creating an environment that would encourage the blue-collar worker to exercise (U.K. Sports Council, 1982a, b). The potential attraction of such an arrangement is a multiplier effect from private investment. A serious disadvantage is that the objective of the brewery is to sell a sedative drug (alcohol) rather than to deliver fitness.

The Needs of Urban Ghettos. In the U.K. the urban riots of Hoxteth and Brixton gave a strong impetus to the establishment of inner-city sport facilities. It was reasoned that if only 1 in 40 of those who were imprisoned could be diverted to community care and 1 in 40 of those in community care could be given a noncriminal means of self-expression, then the construction of sport facilities would be a sound economic investment. In North America, criminal detention now costs up to $70,000 per prisoner per year. Against this must be set the view of one U.S. group that some urban parks actually increase vandalism and the need for police protection (Kavanagh et al., 1973).

Nash (1960) pointed out three possible ways of spending leisure time: (a) ''going to sleep'' in some spectator process, (b) wasting time in social deviancy, and (c) participating in some constructive pursuit. Unfortunately, the depression associated with unemployment and the personal costs of participation encourage (a) and (b) rather than (c). Nevertheless, a need exists to develop adventure-type programs that will offer an alternative to social deviancy and give meaning to the lives of those trapped in an urban jungle of poverty, poor housing, and unemployment (Heaps

& Thorstenson, 1974). Aging factories, schools, docks, and railway yards are being abandoned in city cores, and a considerable potential exists to apply both buildings and released space to the needs of physical activity.

Outdoor Pursuits

Geography and Recreational Demand. The climate and physical geography of the local environment has a major influence upon the demand for and the availability of outdoor recreation.

Usage of distant facilities depends largely upon access roads and vehicle ownership. The price of gasoline is also beginning to limit recreational travel. In England, the Countryside Commission (1978) found that rising fuel prices had curtailed use of the countryside by 51% among those with an annual income of less than $3000, and had curtailed use by 9% among those with an income of more than $24,000. In North America, pump prices of gasoline are currently less than in Britain, particularly if measured relative to disposable income, and to date, fuel costs have had only a minor influence upon the activity patterns of ordinary people.

Relatively few recommendations concerning a desirable scale of outdoor facilities are available. Meyer and Brightbill (1964) proposed building one tennis court per 2000 people across the U.S. An 18-hole municipal golf course was recommended for every 54,000 people, provided that private courses were also available. Murphy et al. (1973) set a similar standard for tennis courts (1/2000), but proposed a much larger number of golf courses (1/3000).

Low-Cost Options. Hiking is attractive as a low-cost source of healthy outdoor activity. Europe has a great advantage over North America with its wide network of foot- and cycle paths. Development of footpaths requires a close linkage between recreation and other forms of social investment. Access to pleasant walking areas should be assured, preferably by fostering public transportation. A good example of this type of initiative is seen in the Viennese subway system, which provides free leaflets illustrating ''Wanderwegen'' (footpaths) with access points at the end of train and bus routes.

Nuisance must be avoided for any private landowners who are involved, whether the property is being used primarily for agriculture, forestry, water cachement, or mineral exploitation. Government should provide and maintain adequate car parking, toilet arrangements, litter disposal, and signposting. In Britain, management agreements covering the operation of such facilities have been established between local authorities and landowners under the provision of the Countryside Act of 1968.

An analysis by Grayson, Sidaway, and Thompson (1975) suggested that 1 acre of parking allowed 18,000 visitors per year at a British Forestry Commission property. The consumer surplus was estimated at a little under 19 cents per visitor-hour, so that the total yield per year was $3367. Against this was set the capital cost of the parking ($5612), paths ($1871), and loss of timber ($748), jointly amortized at $972 • year^{-1}, with a further $561 for maintenance. Consumer surplus thus showed a substantial profit over operating costs.

Modest financial investments in paths, parking lots, shipways, jetties, and clubhouses greatly increase the potential for outdoor pursuits such as climbing, caving, sailing, riding, swimming, and underwater diving. Some sports such as water skiing and hang-gliding attract a substantial number of spectators. Due provision must then be made to accommodate observers as well as enthusiasts.

Environmental Conservation. Due concern must be shown for preservation of the local fauna and flora; for example, excessive recreational use can disrupt natural breeding cycles (Countryside Commission, 1978). In any fragile ecosystem, avoiding permanent environmental damage from cars, motor boats, snowmobiles, and even foot traffic is vital.

Limitations Imposed by Climate. Climate has an enormous impact upon the use of outdoor recreational resources. The building of shallow sandy beaches can extend the swimming season at lake resorts, but at best 3 months usage is likely; often, this is further curtailed by a cold, wet summer. Likewise, investments in field drainage and/or artificial turf extend the potential season for field sports such as soccer, North American football, and field hockey. If summer daytime temperatures are uninvitingly hot for tennis, provision of artificial lighting can allow play to continue in the cooler evening hours.

Lack of snow can be financially disastrous for the operators of cross-country and downhill ski resorts. Again, provision of lighted trails allows maximal use to be made of days when conditions are favorable, while provision of heated shelters and changing rooms encourages continued participation on days that would otherwise be uncomfortably cold.

Role of the Commercial Sector. Public facilities quickly become crowded and detract from the potential pleasure of a beautiful landscape. The private entrepreneur thus has an important role in developing facilities for those who have become attracted to outdoor recreation but wish to pursue this in uncrowded surroundings. Smith and Krutilla (1976) and Shechter and Lucas (1978) have developed mathematical models based on the willingness of individuals to pay for recreational isolation and the likelihood of encountering other travelers. Nevertheless, some forms of wilderness exploration such as the "Outward Bound" scheme function well under public ownership.

Implications for Urban Development. Both Canada and the U.S. continue to allow vast tracts of urban development. Each year the irreversible paving of 1-2 million acres occurs (0.4-0.8 million hectares), mainly over prime agricultural land. The modern megalopolis makes some provision for the outdoor recreation of small children, usually in parkettes linked to primary schools, but the space allocation for adult sport or recreation is far from adequate.

In the U.K., the National Playing Fields Association recommended that for every 1,000 people, 6 acres (2.4 hectares) of land should be dedicated to competitive team games, while the British Sports Council proposed a minimum standard of 3 acres (1.2 hectares) per 1,000 people (U.K. Sports Council, 1976). The latter would provide enough land for 3 closely packed soccer pitches. Pearson (1969) proposed 4 hectares of urban and regional open space per 1,000 people. In the U.S. (Kraus, 1971) the National Recreational Association argued for a more generous total provision of 90 acres (36 hectares) of recreational land per 1,000 people—25 acres (10 hectares) at the municipal and 65 acres (26 hectares) at the state level. The U.S. proposal would require a generous allocation of 240,000 hectares to urban parks, plus 624,000 hectares to state parks, the latter being accessible after no more than 2-3 hrs of traveling.

Applying the British playing field standard to North America, the environmental cost for 300 million people would be 36,000 hectares of land, and with efficient scheduling (4 soccer matches in a day), 26% participation in a team sport such as soccer would be possible. In fact, the participation rate for most sports is much lower than this. In the southeastern part of the U.K., data were collected recently on the number of males, aged 10-44 years, needed to form a single team for various sports; figures were not given for young women, although many of them are now expressing an interest in the same types of activities. Because 150 men were needed to generate a soccer team, a sport field allowance of 1.2 hectares per 1,000 people satisfied the demand for pitches. Even larger numbers of citizens were required to generate an interest in other sports (400 males of similar age were required to form a cricket team, 1,600 to form a rugger team, and over 8,000 to form a field hockey team).

Similar problems of low-participation rates arise when sport-specific playing areas are established in North America. However, the further complication of a short playing season for many outdoor activities exists because of extremes of heat or cold.

A more radical approach to urban planning builds physical activity into the normal day, sometimes at substantial savings to the developer

(Fabun, 1971). Cluster zoning of housing, shops, and industry allows the majority of journeys to be made on foot or by cycle. The cost of foot- and cycle paths is naturally much lower than either roads or subway lines. Again, the wholehearted adoption of this European concept is helped by design features that temper extremes of climate. Trees provide summer shade and act as barriers to noise and air pollution, while in winter suitable grading avoids the accumulation of water and ice on paths.

Conclusions

The cost of programs and facilities that enhance physical fitness varies widely, depending upon the luxury of what is provided and the efficiency of scheduling. Exercise testing by a physician could prove to be a costly start-up feature ($100 or more per participant), but this would be unnecessary for healthy adults who are proposing a gradual increase of physical activity. A rough guide to an appropriate prescription can be obtained by self-testing (Home Fitness Kit, $10 per family), while more precise prescriptions can be provided by a paramedical professional ($10.44 per test with heavy usage of the test facility).

Industrial exercise facilities are generally more cost-effective than community operations. Estimates of the expense vary with the completeness of accounting (e.g., whether or not allowance is made for space rental and occupancy charges), but with 20% program participation a range of $80-150 per worker-year may be assumed.

Public parks within a city are an important general amenity and add to property values, but they often get rather limited use as a source of physical activity. A conservation-type regional park is a much lower cost investment: An example of $108 per user-year, or $21.60 per citizen-year is cited. The main disadvantages of the regional park are travel costs and a short season for such pursuits as outdoor swimming and cross-country skiing.

The cost of indoor facilities depends not only on luxury and scheduling, but also on land prices and the amount of parking that is provided. Capital costs could be greatly reduced by the control of urban land speculation and the building of a sufficient number of facilities to allow access by foot or by bicycle. The impact of excessive land prices is even greater for some outdoor team sports such as soccer and football.

Personal activities such as walking and jogging all lead to significant expenditures by the active individual. Typical costs include clothing, footwear, timing devices, food, and travel to meets. Many argue that one important emphasis in future urban planning should be the facilitation of self-propelled transportation. In addition to the health benefits of walking and cycling, large expenditures on roads and subway systems would be avoided.

Medical supervision of exercise programs is not cost-effective; a more appropriate tactic for increasing the safety of exercise classes is widespread public education in techniques of cardiopulmonary resuscitation. Moreover, the risks of physical activity in an ostensibly healthy adult are quite low; it should be possible to insure against a cardiac catastrophe during a submaximal stress test for about 1.3 cents. Unless the level of competition is very intense, sport injuries are also only a minor concern, leading to absenteeism expenses of about $5.12 per worker-year and treatment costs of $0.23-0.90 per worker-year.

Active recreation creates environmental pressures through the need for access roads, land devoted to facilities and parking, and degradation of wilderness areas. Such costs are difficult to value, but can be a severe problem for crowded European countries. Care is needed to preserve both fragile ecosystems and prime agricultural land. Much of the necessary space for a more active population could be found in de-industrialized wasteland. A major need exists for active recreation to counter social deviancy in the decaying cores of large cities, and, given the high costs of detention ($70,000 per prisoner-year), the impact of fitness programing upon social deviancy merits more careful evaluation. Finally, more thought must be directed to cost-effective methods of extending the user-season for outdoor facilities throughout the climatic extremes of summer and winter.

chapter 7

Toward a Balance Sheet

All the data available nationally are inaccurate and incomplete in varying ways. (Rodgers, 1978)

This final chapter will highlight several ethical issues involved in the active promotion of health and fitness. It will also define areas of research priority and will present an interim balance sheet for a more active society.

Ethical Issues

It has already been noted that the support of governmental programs ultimately tends to be determined by a combination of pressure groups, marginal constituents, and the general electorate rather than by some absolute ethical standard espoused by an individual government department. In the area of health, economics is not always the reason for success or failure of a policy. The imagination of the general public is often captured by skillfully publicized dramatic acute-care interventions such as heart and liver transplants. Enthusiasm is generated for the "miracles" of modern medicine, with little regard for either cost/benefit ratio or cost-effectiveness (Hetherington & Calderone, 1983). Nevertheless, the government has a responsibility to lay ethical problems clearly before the electorate and give as accurate a picture as possible of the financial consequences of various alternative policies.

The active promotion of physical fitness raises several important ethical issues, each with its particular budgetary implications. Should fitness be promoted while many of the supposed benefits such as protection against ischemic heart disease are strong inferences rather than rigidly proven scientific facts? If fitness is to be promoted, how far does the ordinary citizen have the right to remain unfit? If fitness and health promotion cannot be fully justified on cost/benefit grounds, how far should such initiatives continue relative to other governmental priorities such as defense, provision for the elderly and unemployed, education, or treatment of overt diseases? Lastly, is it most appropriate to concentrate promotional efforts upon changing the lifestyle of the individual, or should prime attention be directed to those features of the environment that influence personal activity?

Extent of Proof

P.O. Åstrand has commented that he would have more concern about the health of a person who did not exercise than one who did. This seems to be a fair assessment of the available epidemiological evidence; an increase of physical activity would probably reduce the risk of ischemic heart disease by at least 50% and would become a beneficial influence upon a number of other medical conditions. Thus no medical grounds exist for objecting to the promotion of an increased level of physical activity.

There have been some calculations of the cost of proving the "exercise hypothesis" to the satisfaction of a skeptical statistician. Taylor, Parkin, Blackburn, and Keys (1966) estimated that even if a high-risk population was recruited, the expense of a controlled experiment would amount to the equivalent of $123 million. Moreover, the proof would remain relatively unsatisfactory because of a high rate of dropouts from the experimental category and some contamination of controls with an interest in exercise. Scope remains for examining other more cost-effective methods of answering the important question of whether activity influences health. Possibly health experience could be correlated prospectively with activity patterns and fitness levels as determined from a succession of national fitness surveys, or possibly the case-control method already used by Morris et al. (1973) could be exploited more fully.

Right to Remain Unfit

Authority for choice was discussed briefly in chapter 1. While a lawyer might argue for the basic human right to remain unfit and unhealthy, the evidence presented suggests that insistence upon this right imposes a substantial fiscal burden for such items as health care costs on other members of society.

Perhaps people are entitled to remain unfit *only if* they are prepared to meet the additional health costs incurred by the exploitation of this right. Further study of differential health insurance premiums is desirable. The main argument against this policy is that some people might (for various legitimate reasons) be unable to improve their personal fitness. The analysis should make a full assessment of such issues as (a) the costs of assessing compliance with a basic exercise prescription, (b) the costs of assessing reasons for noncompliance, and (c) the increased cost of collecting differential premiums.

Governmental Priorities

Setting governmental expenditures one against the other is beyond the scope of this book, although the sums of money involved are so large that the necessary decisions become a major ethical issue.

The cost-effectiveness of exercise programs can nevertheless be weighed against statistics for other health promotion tactics. Smoking cessation programs, recently costed at $240-600 per successful withdrawal (Brennan, 1982a), could represent a more favorable investment of tax dollars than activity programming because the expense is of a once-only nature. On the other hand, some reports suggest that relatively few people are helped by formal smoking withdrawal clinics (Shephard & LaBarre, 1976). The treatment of hypertension costs $180-240 per year per patient (Kristein, 1982) and, given a rather poor compliance with prescribed medications, the expense of operating a program for those with high blood pressure is at least as great as that of providing regular physical activity classes. Moreover, the risk of complications from the use of hypotensive drugs is substantial, while the matching spectrum of benefits is quite limited.

Careful accounting ultimately seems likely to establish a favorable cost/benefit ratio for enhanced physical activity, so that the difficult task of comparing cost-effectiveness with other possible preventive tactics may not be necessary. If exercise does lead to cost savings, the main question for government then becomes, What is the maximum investment it can usefully make in physical activity programing? Plainly, at some point further expenditures induce no further gains of fitness. However, this point probably has not yet been reached in terms of either promotion of physical activity or the provision of programs and facilities. For example, the current budgets of such agencies as the U.S. President's Council on Fitness and Canadian fitness promotion agencies remain miniscule relative to private spending on the advertising of such items as alcohol and cigarettes. Likewise, some of the more aggressive operators of private fitness clubs find it useful to allocate as much as a third of their revenues to the promotion of facilities and programs.

Personal Responsibility

The issue of personal versus societal responsibility for fitness was broached in chapter 3. In the U.S. there has been little debate that "Health promotion places the emphasis on the individual *where it belongs''* (Novelli & Ziska, 1982, p. 21). The Canadian government has not made quite such an unequivocal statement, but to date the main thrust of its efforts has been toward securing a change in personal behavior (World Health Forum, 1981; Landry et al., 1982). Twelve of 23 current health promotion tactics seek to induce an increase of physical activity (Lalonde, 1974).

It has been suggested that regulatory mechanisms are "conspicuously unsuccessful''in altering the attitudes that determine individual life-style. Nevertheless, the cost-effectiveness of a societal versus a personal approach to fitness has yet to be measured carefully. Discussions with union representatives suggest that the current emphasis on personal rather than corporate behavior may present some barrier to involvement of the targeted blue-collar population. The type of argument is best exemplified by attempts to foster a healthy life-style in a paint factory that has used a large quantity of asbestos in its manufacturing processes—the introduction of a smoking withdrawal program is then resisted by union representatives because it is perceived as an attempt to shift responsibility for asbestosis from management to the worker (who may be a continuing or former smoker). Likewise, a fitness program may be viewed as a means of shifting the blame for back injuries from a badly designed loading bay to a lack of physical strength.

A further concern is that undue emphasis upon individual action has the effect of widening the gap in health between the upper- and lower-socioeconomic strata (Mullen, 1981; McGinnis, 1982). This dilemma can be alleviated somewhat if government assumes the responsibility of providing knowledge, facilities, and financial support to encourage the desired actions by poorer members of society (Etzioni, 1978).

The essential ethical problem is the individual's right to remain unfit (Pellegrino, 1981). If society has conditioned a blue-collar worker, an unemployed teenager, or a housewife to undertake little deliberate physical activity from an early age (Allison & Coburn, 1981), is it then fair to apply such sanctions as differential health premiums to those who are unfit? Equally, should employees such as police or firefighters be placed on leave without pay if they fail to maintain certain minimum standards of personal condition? In practice a consensus on this, as on other important questions, will probably be reached on political rather than ethical grounds.

Research Priorities

Two bases may be suggested for establishing research priorities in the area of cost/benefit analyses—currently perceived governmental priorities, and policy sectors with a large potential cost/benefit ratio.

Evaluation of Governmental Programs

It is arguable that government has already given much thought to ethically acceptable and politically realistic options, so that cost-effectiveness and cost/benefit analysis should be applied specifically to items where expenditures are currently high. The main obstacle to this tactic is that program costs are already fairly well-established, while benefits are dispersed over a wide range of effects in governmental, entrepreneurial, and personal sectors. If such a tactic is indeed to be adopted, cost-effectiveness seems to be a more appropriate basis of judgment than cost/benefit analysis. Tasks that remain include the following:

1. An overall criterion of effectiveness should be determined. (The choice might be between a measure of behavior, such as a minimum recommended activity level versus a measure of attained fitness such as a combination of aerobic power, body fat, muscular strength, and flexibility.)
2. Assessment of the percentages of white-collar and blue-collar groups who can be brought to an adequate standard of personal activity or physical fitness through
   (a) selected promotional tactics and the cost per individual convert of the various approaches to lifestyle modification.
   (b) the provision of various types of programs and facilities. Specific comparisons are needed between the merits of employee fitness programs, employee sport programs, municipal indoor and outdoor recreational programs, and regional recreation programs. More detailed analysis should also look at individual pursuits within each of these environments. Again, all data should be expressed as a cost per fitness convert.
   (c) investment in spectator sport (construction of domed stadia for commercial franchises and support of state or provincial, national, and international competitions). Again, all data should be expressed as a cost per fitness convert.

Sectors Possibly Having Large Cost/Benefit Ratios

Personal benefits that merit more accurate assessment include the following:

Enhancement of Academic Learning. The supposed opportunity cost of required physical education has been a major stumbling block to the upgrading of school physical activity programs, especially at the primary school level (where socialization into sport is most readily achieved). The encouraging finding that required physical education actually enhances academic learning (chapter 2) merits early confirmation.

Life Satisfaction. A second personal benefit from regular physical activity is an increase of life satisfaction. More research is needed on the extent of changes in life satisfaction with participation in various types of programs, considering the impact upon various target groups, methods of costing, and implications for the functional performance of the individual.

Medical Care Demands. The reduced demand for both acute and chronic health care is apparently a major benefit of enhanced physical activity (chapter 2). The upper limit of such benefit could probably be established by a cross-sectional and retrospective analysis of health-care usage, classified by activity history. More precise limits could be set by a case-control approach that matches active and inactive subjects for confounding variables such as social class and cigarette and alcohol consumption.

Sociocultural Benefits.

Compliance. Key variables in almost all calculations of costs and benefits are the participation rates of the target population and the manner in which the individuals' participation is modified by promotional and program tactics. Further work is necessary to clarify how far the present level of participation could be increased by greater corporate or governmental expenditures. Examining what types of programming might extend both recruitment and compliance is also necessary.

Unemployment. Preliminary analyses of the impact of physical activity programs upon regional unemployment seem most encouraging (chapter 3). However, scope is available for more detailed examination; the number of jobs created for a $1M investment in active recreation should be tested and compared to other labor-intensive policies.

Industrial Benefits. Although absenteeism is perhaps the most easily measured variable, larger economic benefits may be anticipated from the impact of personal fitness upon the quality and the quantity of production and from a reduction of turnover among physically active employees (chapter 5). Methods are needed to measure productivity more precisely in both blue- and white-collar employment, relating changes in this variable to enhancement of physical fitness.

Geriatric Benefits.

Independence. An extension of the period of independent living would be a major social benefit and would lead to significant practical consequences in terms of the costs of residential care (chapter 5). Further research into the key factors responsible for institutionalization and the extent to which such limiting circumstances can be deferred through an increase of personal physical activity is needed.

Support Costs. A detailed accounting of support costs for the active versus the inactive senior citizen is required in order to explore the bogey that an active person may live longer and thus become a greater financial burden upon society.

Program Costs

While the governmental costs of existing programs are established fairly clearly, data on the expenditures that would be necessary in order to reach current target groups such as blue-collar workers, the unemployed, single mothers, and social deviants is needed. An additional need is further data on (a) the willingness of the population to meet a part of the fiscal costs of fitness through such measures as admission fees and (b) the impact upon participation of opportunity costs such as the need to travel to a distant facility.

Conclusions: An Interim Balance Sheet

We may conclude by drawing up a balance sheet for the personal, private, and governmental sectors of the economy. The government must be concerned not only with its immediate fiscal problems but also with the costs and benefits experienced by individuals and private corporations. Not only is the government responsible to those it serves, but also, in the long-term, the happiness and productivity of any nation determine the amount of money that will be available to government for its future programs. Thus no apology is necessary for introducing all three sectors of the economy into our balance sheet. Dollar figures are not included (Table 7.1), although details for many items have been cited earlier in the text.

Table 7.1 Costs and Benefits of Enhanced Physical Activity

Costs	Benefits
Personal	
Food	Better intake of nutrients/vitamins
Clothing	Reduced expenditure on alcohol/tobacco/drugs, other forms
Equipment	of recreation, dress clothing
Admission fees	New experiences
Travel/lodging	Meaning for age of leisure/employment
Time	Reduced industrial and domestic injury
Injury	Improvements of perceived health, reduction of acute and
Death	chronic disease, enhanced quality of geriatric life
	Control of alcohol/tobacco/drug dependency/less passive
	smoking and fires
	Improved personal appearance
	Enhanced property values
	Fewer problems from social deviancy
Private Sector	
Exercise facilities	Worker satisfaction
Medical supervision,	Enhanced productivity
exercise personnel	Reduced turnover and absenteeism
Time	Reduced industrial injuries
Sport injuries	Reduced health insurance premiums
	Enhanced company image
	Enhanced employment/economic growth
	Entrepreneurial opportunities
	Enhanced property values
Government	
Fitness promotion	Reduced hospital and health-care costs
Exercise facilities	Reduced social deviancy (vandalism, law enforcement, detention)
Recreational workers	Reduced geriatric dependency
Land acquisition	Enhanced employment
Infrastructure (roads,	Economic stimulation/increased tax base
mass transit, etc.)	Enhanced environment
	Improved balance of payments
	Worker benefits in government-controlled enterprises (as
	noted above for private sector companies)
	Military fitness

The costs and benefits incurred by an active individual have been discussed in chapter 2. Expenses are incurred for the purchase of additional food, but this helps to ensure a balanced intake of vitamins and essential nutrients. The costs of recreational clothing and equipment are offset by a decrease in other nonessential purchases—passive recreation, dress clothing, alcohol, tobacco, and drugs. Such changes in the use of disposable income have a beneficial effect upon personal health. Travel and lodging are optional costs associated with some types of active recreation and also carry the opportunity dividend of new experiences. A substantial amount of time can be claimed by the pursuit of fitness, particularly if facilities are distant from the place of residence; however, most North Americans have long periods of disposable time, and the development of meaningful and active leisure pursuits will assume ever-increasing importance as full-time employment opportunities diminish. Moreover, the labor-intensive nature of many types of active recreation has the potential to increase employment by 5-6%.

Exercise may cause injury and even death, but this small risk must be set against a reduced long-term risk of injury in both industry and the home; instead, exercise offers an improved perceived health, a lesser risk of both acute and chronic diseases, and an enhanced quality of retirement years. Dependency upon alcohol, tobacco, and drugs may be cured, and less hazards from fire and passive exposure to cigarette smoke will result. Personal appearance will be enhanced, property values may rise, and fewer problems will be encountered from social deviancy.

The main expense to the private sector of the economy is the cost of developing and maintaining any in-house exercise facilities and providing necessary program supervision. Some time may be lost to normal production because employees attend exercise tests and programs or devise promotional material such as newsletters for fitness classes. Flexible scheduling of working hours is necessary to obtain maximum use of an exercise facility. Lastly, minor expenses (time loss, workmen's compensation) may be incurred from sport-related injuries. On the positive side of the ledger are increased worker satisfaction and gains in both the quantity and the quality of industrial output. Turnover and absenteeism are reduced, and the risk of industrial injury decreases. Medical insurance premiums may also be lowered because the workers are sick less frequently. Less direct benefits include an enhancement of company image, a stimulation of the general economy, entrepreneurial opportunities for the development of programs and facilities in the recreational field, and enhancement of property values secondary to recreational development.

Government faces costs for both the promotion of fitness and the provision of programs. Land must be acquired; an infrastructure of services must be installed; facilities must be built, equipped, and staffed; and due allowance must be made for depreciation of both facilities and equipment. Direct benefits to government include reduced hospital and medical costs, reduced social deviancy (with an impact upon vandalism, law enforcement, and detention costs), reduced geriatric dependency (and thus a reduced need for welfare and make-work programs), economic stimulation (enlarging the tax base), environmental improvement (particularly through the development of new areas of parkland), an improved balance of international payments (more inward movement of tourists, less extraterritorial recreation), benefits to government-controlled enterprises (as in the private sector), and improved fitness for national defense.

References

Åberg, H., & Hedstrand, H. (1976). Treatment of hypertension in middle-aged men: A feasibility study in the community. *Clinical Science and Molecular Medicine,* **51,** S975-S995.

Ableson, J., Paddon, P., & Strohmenger, C. (1983). *Perspectives on health* (Occasional Paper, 82-540E). Ottawa: Ministry of Supply & Services.

Activity Research Associates. (1981). *Low active adults—Who they are, how to reach them.* Toronto: Ontario Ministry of Culture and Recreation.

Adachi, N. (1978). *Job redesign for the Japanese older workers* (Abstract). 11th International Congress of Gerontology, Tokyo.

Alchian, A.A., & Kessell, R.A. (1977). Competition, monopoly and the pursuit of money. In *Economic forces at work* (pp. 151-176). Indianapolis: Liberty Press.

Allen, R.F. (1977). A cultural-based approach to the improvement of health practice. *Proceedings of the 13th Meeting of Society for Prospective Medicine & Health Education Resources* (pp. 11-14).

Allison, K., & Coburn, D. (1981). *Blue collar workers and physical activity.* Toronto: Ontario Ministry of Culture and Recreation.

Anderson, R.W. (1975). Estimating the recreation benefit from large inland reservoirs. In G.A. Searle (Ed.), *Recreational economics and analysis* (pp. 75-88). Harlow, Essex: Longman.

Anderson, T.W., & Halliday, M.L. (1979). The male epidemic: 50 years of ischaemic heart disease. *Public Health (London),* **93,** 163-172.

Andrevsky, J.H. (1982, December). Corporate sweat. *The Runner.* pp. 40-44.

Andrisani, P.J. (1978). *Job dissatisfaction among older men: Some evidence and implications for job redesign and retraining programs for older workers* (Abstract). 11th International Congress of Gerontology, Tokyo.

Antonini, F. (1971). Some reflections on the anthropology and biology of work. In J.A. Huet (Ed.), *Work & aging* (pp. 13-20). Paris: International Centre of Social Gerontology.

Arrowsmith, G. (1979). Sports usage and membership at a large urban leisure complex: Billingham Forum. (*Research Working Papers,* **17**, 1-12). London: Sports Council.

Atchley, R.C. (1971). Retirement and leisure participation: Continuity or crisis? *Gerontologist,* **12**, 13.

Atchley, R.C. (1977). *The social forces in later life* (2nd ed.). Belmont, CA: Wadsworth.

Atherley, G.R.C., Gale, R.W., & Drummond, M.F. (1976). An approach to the financial evaluation of occupational health services. *Journal of Social and Occupational Medicine,* **26**, 21-30.

Atkinson, J., & Collins, M.F. (1980). The impact of neighbouring sports and leisure centres. (*Research Working Papers,* **18**, 1-12). London: Sports Council.

Aubry, J.P., & Fleurent, D. (1980). Simulation analysis of a model based on the life-cycle hypothesis (*Technical Report,* HQ1061 B 413 1977). Ottawa, Canada: Bank of Canada.

Back, K.W. (1969). The ambiguity of retirement. In E.W. Busse & E. Pfeiffer (Eds.), *Behaviour and adaptation in late life* (pp. 78-98). Boston: Little Brown.

Bailey, D.A., Shephard, R.J., & Mirwald, R. (1976). Validation of a self-administered home test of cardio-respiratory fitness. *Canadian Journal of Applied Sport Sciences,* **1**, 67-78.

Bailey, D.A., Shephard, R.J., Mirwald, R.L., & Weese, R. (1974). Current levels of cardio-respiratory fitness. *Canadian Medical Association Journal,* **111**, 25-30.

Banister, E. (1978). Health, fitness and productivity. In E.W. Banister (Ed.), *Human performance in business and industry* (pp. 9-21). Burnaby, British Columbia: Simon Fraser University Press.

Bannister, R. (1972). Sport, physical recreation and the national health. *British Medical Journal,* **(iv)**, 711-715.

Barhad, B. (1979). Physical activity in modern history. *Physiologie,* **16**, 117-122.

Barnard, R.J., & Anthony, D.F. (1980). Effect of health maintenance programs on Los Angeles City firefighters. *Journal of Occupational Medicine,* **22**, 667-669.

Beck, R.N. (1982). IBM's plan for life: Towards a comprehensive health care strategy. *Health Education Quarterly,* **9** (Suppl.), 55-60.

Bellefleur, M. (1976). Budget des Jeux de '76 aurait pu financer 10,000 piscines: Été hiver Olympic mania. *Recreation Canada,* **34**, 44-45.

Bellina, L., Savalla, G., Caruso, C., & Matracia, S. (1980). Modifications of peripheral white cells after short term stress in football players. In L. Vecchiet (Ed.), *1st International Congress on Sports Medicine applied to football* (pp. 291-298). Rome: D. Guanella.

Bennett, B.L., Howell, M.L., & Simri, U. (1983). *Comparative physical education and sport* (pp. 1-283). Philadelphia: Lea & Febiger.

Bennett, J.E., & Krasny, J. (1981). Health care and Canada. In D. Coburn, C. D'Arcy, P. New, & G. Torrance (Eds.), *Health and Canadian society* (pp. 40-66). Toronto: Fitzhenry & Whiteside.

Berger, E. (1983). *Recreation—A changing society's economic grant.* Toronto: Ministry of Tourism and Recreation.

Berkman, L.F., & Syme, S.L. (1979). Social networks, host resistance and mortality. A nine year follow-up study of Alameda County residents. *American Journal of Epidemiology* , **109**, 186-204.

Berl, W.G., & Halpin, B.M. (1978, December). *Human fatalities from unwanted fires* (pp. 1-64). Washington, DC: U.S. Department of Commerce. (National Bureau of Standards Publication 79-168)

Berry, R.E., & Boland, J.P. (1977). *The economic cost of alcohol abuse.* New York: Collier Macmillan.

Betts, J.R. (1974). *America's sporting heritage 1850-1950* (pp. 77-78). Reading, MA: Addison Wesley.

Beverfeldt, E. (1971). Psychic behavior of the worker facing old age. In J.A. Huet (Ed.), *Work and aging* (pp. 135-146). Paris: International Centre of Social Gerontology.

Bidgood R. (1972). Raising finance for recreation facilities. *Parks and Sports Grounds,* **38**, 141-144.

Bierton, R.C.J. (1974). *The recreational carrying capacity of the countryside* (Occasional Publications. Vol. 11). Stafford, United Kingdom: Keele University Library.

Birch, J.G. (1971). *Indoor Sports Centres.* Study 1. London: Her Majesty's Stationery Office for Sports Council.

Bischoff, J., & Maldaner, K. (1980). *Kulturindustrie und ideologie.* Hamburg: VSA Verlag.

Bjurstrom, L.A., & Alexiou, N.G. (1978). A program of heart disease prevention for public employees. *Journal of Occupational Medicine,* **20**, 521-531.

Blair, S., Blair, A., Howe, H., Russell, P., Rosenberg, M., & Parker, G. (1980). Leisure time physical activity and job performance. *Research Quarterly,* **51**, 718-723.

Borkan, G.A., & Norris, A.H. (1980). Biological age in adulthood: Comparison of active and inactive U.S. males. *Human Biology, 52,* 787-802.

Brennan, A.J.J. (1982a). Health promotion: What's in it for business and industry? *Health Education Quarterly, 9* (Suppl.), 9-19.

Brennan, A.J.J. (1982b). Health promotion, health education and prevention at Metropolitan Insurance Companies. *Health Education Quarterly, 9* (Suppl.), 49-54.

Breslow, L., & Enstrom, J.E. (1980). Persistence of health habits and their relation to mortality. *Preventive Medicine, 9,* 469-483.

Briggs, T. (1975, February). Industry starts to take fitness into the plan. *Executive, 17*(2), 25.

British Medical Journal Ed. (1974). Smoking and colds. *British Medical Journal,* **(iii)**, 594.

Brocklehurst, J.C. (1973). Geriatric services and the day hospital. In J.C. Brocklehurst (Ed.), *Textbook of geriatric medicine and gerontology* (pp. 673-691). Edinburgh: Churchill-Livingstone.

Brooke, N. (1979). Contribution of retired persons to society—The Australian scene. In H. Orimo, K. Shimada, M. Iriki, & D. Maeda (Eds.), *Recent advances in gerontology* (pp. 379-380). Amsterdam: Excerpta Medica.

Brown, J.R. (1972). *Manual lifting and related fields* (An annotated bibliography). Toronto: Labour Safety Council, Ontario Dept. of Labour.

Brunner, D., Manelis, G., Modan, M., & Levin, S. (1974). Physical activity at work and the incidence of myocardial infarction, angina pectoris and death due to ischemic heart disease. *Journal of Chronic Diseases, 27,* 217-233.

Built Environment Research Group. (1978). *Sport in a jointly provided centre. Study 14.* London: The Sports Council.

Butson, P. (1983). *The financing of sport in the United Kingdom.* London: The Sports Council.

Butz, W.P., & Ward, M.P. (1978). The emergence of countercyclical U.S. fertility. *American Economic Review, 69,* 318-328.

Byrd, R. (1976, December). Impact of physical fitness on police performance. *Police Chief,* pp. 30-32.

Campbell, J. (1979). Facility considerations in employee fitness programming. In R. Wanzel (Ed.), *Employee fitness—The how to* (pp. 71-79). Toronto: Ministry of Culture and Recreation.

Canada Fitness Survey. (1983). *Fitness and aging.* Ottawa: Fitness and Amateur Sport.

Canada Health Survey. (1982). *The health of Canadians* (Paper 82-538E). Ottawa: Statistics Canada.

Cappon, D. (1983, March/April). Searching for health and welfare. *Policy Options*, pp. 27-30.

Carter, R., & Wanzel, R. (1975). Measuring recreation's effect on productivity. *Recreation Management*, **18**(6), 42-47.

Centre Internationale de Securité. (1962). *International Occupational Safety and Health Information Centre*. Information Sheet 3. Geneva: ILO.

Chambers, L.W. (1982). Health program review in Canada: Measurement of health status. *Canadian Journal of Public Health*, **73**, 26-34.

Changing Times. (1974, April). P. 16.

Chappell, N.L. (1980). Social policy and the elderly. In V. Marshall (Ed.), *Aging in Canada* (pp. 35-42). Toronto: Fitzhenry & Whiteside.

The Chartered Institute of Public Finance and Accountancy. (1979). *Leisure and recreation statistics 1979-80 estimates*. London: Author.

Cheraskin, E., & Ringsdorf, W.M. (1973). Predictive medicine. X. Physical activity. *Journal of the American Geriatric Society*, **19**, 969-973.

Chevalier, N., Garnier, C., & Girard, A. (1983). Profile et motivations des skieurs de fond. *Canadian Journal of Applied Sport Sciences*, **8**, 227.

Chisholm, D.M. (1975). The role of the health professional in employee fitness programmes (direct and supportive). In S. Keir (Ed.), *Employee physical fitness in Canada* (pp. 44-47). Ottawa: Health and Welfare Canada.

Chisholm, D.M. (1977). Occupational health—A priority and a challenge. *Canadian Journal of Public Health*, **68**, 189-191.

Chisholm, D.M., Collis, M.L., Kulak, L.L., Davenport, W., & Gruber, N. (1975). Physical activity readiness. *British Columbia Medical Journal*, **17**, 375-378.

Chown, I. (1962). Adaptability to technological change. [Cited by M. Roth.] In International Labour Office, Report of the Director General (Ed.), *Mental health problems of aging and the aged with some comments on the role of World Health and other international organizations*. Part I. Old people—Work and retirement. Geneva: International Labour Office.

Cicchetti, C.J. (1973). *Forecasting recreation in the United States. An economic review of methods and applications to plan for the required environmental resources*. Lexington, MA: D.C. Heath.

Cillari, E., Gargano, M.R., Bellavia, A., & Matracia, S. (1980). Effect of short-term stress on lymphoid cell sub-populations in trained football players. In L. Vecchiet (Ed.), *1st International Congress on Sports Medicine applied to football* (pp. 299-305). Rome: D. Guanella.

Clark, R., Kreps, J., & Spengler, J. (1978). Economics of aging: A survey. *Journal of Economic Literature, 16,* 919-962.

Clawson, M., & Knetsch, J.L. (1966). *Economics of outdoor recreation*. Baltimore: Johns Hopkins Press.

Clement, W. (1975). *The Canadian corporate elite*. Toronto: McClelland & Stewart.

Collings, G.H. (1982). Managing the health of the employee. *Journal of Occupational Medicine, 24,* 15-17.

Collis, M. (1977). *Employee fitness*. Minister of State for Fitness and Amateur Sport, Health and Welfare. Ottawa: Queen's Printer.

Comfort, A. (1973). Theories of aging. In J.C. Brocklehurst (Ed.), *Textbook of geriatric medicine & gerontology* (pp. 46-59). Edinburgh: Churchill Livingstone.

Comfort, A. (1979). *The biology of senescence* (3rd ed.). New York: Elsevier.

Condon, J. (1977, October). Executive sweat. *Women Sports*, pp. 20-23. [Cited by R.S. Wanzel, 1979]

Conference Board. (1972). *Road maps of industry—Leisure*. Ottawa: Author.

Cooper, K.H. (1968). A means of assessing maximal oxygen intake. *Journal of the American Medical Association, 203,* 201-204.

Cooper, K.H. (1970). Guidelines for managing the exercising patient. *Journal of the American Medical Association, 211,* 1663-1667.

Cooper, K.H., Pollock, M.L., Martin, R.P., White, S.R., Linnerud, A.C., & Jackson, A. (1976). Physical fitness levels and selected coronary risk factors. A cross-sectional study. *Journal of the American Medical Association, 236,* 166-169.

Coopers & Lybrand Associates. (1981). *Sharing does work. The economic and social costs and benefits of joint and direct sports provision* (No. 21). London: Sports Council Study.

Coronio, G., & Muret, J.P. (1973). *Loisir. Du Mythe aux réalités*. Paris: Centre de Récherche d'Urbanisme.

Corrigan, D.L. (1980). Effect of habitual exercise on total health as reflected by non-accidental insurance claims. Action: *American Association of Fitness Directors in Business & Industry Journal, 3,* 7-8.

Council of Executive Directors. (1983). *Corporate sponsors and amateur sport: An unbeatable team*. Ottawa: Brief by Council of Executive Directors at the National Sport and Recreation Centre.

Countryside Commission. (1977). Recreation cost-benefit analysis. In *Leisure and the countryside* (pp. 1-26). London: Author.

Countryside Commission. (1978). *The countryside recreation research advisory group conference, 1978*. London: Janssen Services.

Cox, M., Shephard, R.J., & Corey, P. (1981). Influence of an employee fitness programme upon fitness, productivity and absenteeism. *Ergonomics*, **24**, 795-806.

Cox, M., Shephard, R.J., & Corey, P. (1982). *Physical activity and alienation in the work place*. Paper presented at North American Symposium on Sociology of Sport. Toronto.

Cozens, F.W., & Stumpf, F.S. (1953). *Sports in American life*. Chicago: University of Chicago Press.

Crompton, J.L. (1976). Planning. Problems of provision and planning for leisure. In J.T. Haworth & M.A. Smith (Eds.), *An inter-disciplinary study in theory, education and planning*. Princeton, NJ: Princeton Book Company.

Culture Statistics. (1978). *Culture Statistics Service Bulletin Catalog 87-001*. Ottawa: Statistics Canada.

Danaher, B.G. (1980). Smoking cessation programs in occupational settings. *Public Health Reports*, **95**, 149-157.

Danielson, R., & Danielson, K. (1982). *Exercise program effects on productivity of forestry firefighters*. Toronto: Ontario Ministry of Tourism and Recreation.

Darnley, F. (1975). Adjustment to retirement—Integrity or despair? *Family Coordinator*, **24**, 217.

Dauriac, C.M. (1982). Sport and the voluntary non-profit sector of the economy—A Franco-American comparison. In *Proceedings, 2nd International Seminar on Comparative Physical Education and Sport*, (pp. 57-77). Halifax.

Davies, G.W. (1977). Macro-economic effects of immigration: Evidence from CANDIDE, TRACE and RDX-2. *Canadian Public Policy*, **3**, 299-306.

DeCarlo, T.J. (1974). Recreation participation patterns and successful aging. *Journal of Gerontology*, **29**, 416-422.

Decker, D.L. (1980). *Social gerontology. An introduction to the dynamics of aging*. Boston: Little, Brown & Co.

Delarue, N.C. (1973). A study in smoking withdrawal. *Canadian Journal of Public Health, 64*, S5-S19.

Denton, F., Feaver, C., & Spencer, B. (1980). *The future population and labour force of Canada: Projections to the year 2051*. Ottawa: Economic Council of Canada.

Denton, F., & Spencer, B. (1980a). Canada's population and labour force. Past, present and future. In V.W. Marshall (Ed.), *Aging in Canada. Social perspectives* (pp. 10-26). Toronto: Fitzhenry & Whiteside.

Denton, F., & Spencer, B. (1980b). Health care costs when the population changes. In V.W. Marshall (Ed.), *Aging in Canada. Social perspectives* (pp. 232-247). Toronto: Fitzhenry & Whiteside.

Department of Health and Social Security. (1977). *Prevention and health*. London: Her Majesty's Stationery Office.

Dodov, N., Ploshtakov, P., Patcharazov, V., & Nilolova, L. (1975). Active sport as a factor for decreasing diseases with temporary working incapability among industrial workers. In A.H. Toyne (Ed.), *Proceedings of 20th World Congress in Sports Medicine* (p. 231). Melbourne: Australian Sports Medicine Federation.

Donoghue, S. (1977). The correlation between physical fitness, absenteeism and work performance. *Canadian Journal of Public Health, 68*, 201-203.

Dowd, J.W. (1975). Aging as exchange: A preface to theory. *Journal of Gerontology, 30*(5), 584-594.

Draper, J.E. (1967). *Work attitudes and retirement adjustment*. Madison, WI: University of Wisconsin Bureau of Business Research and Service.

Drummond, M.F. (1980). *Principles of economic appraisal in health care*. Oxford, United Kingdom: Oxford University Press.

Drummond, M.F., & Mooney, G.H. (1982). Part II—Financing health care. *British Medical Journal, 285*, 1101-1103.

Duare, R.B., & Kreuter, M.W. (1981). Reinforcing the case for health promotion. *Family and Community Health, 2*, 103-119.

Duffield, B.S. (1975). The nature of recreational travel space. In G.A. Searle (Ed.), *Recreational economics and analysis* (pp. 15-35). Harlow, Essex: Longman.

Duggar, C.V., & Swengros, G.V. (1969). The design of physical activity programs for industry. *Journal of Occupational Medicine, 11*, 322-329.

Dumazedier, J., & Imbert, M. (1964). *Espace et loisir dans la societé française d'hier et de demain*. Paris: Centre de Récherche d'Urbanisme.

Durbeck, D.C., Heinzelmann, F., Schachter, J., Haskell, W.L., Payne, G.H., Moxley, R.T., Nemiroff, M., Limoncelli, D., Arnoldi, L., & Fox, S. (1972). The National Aeronautics and Space Administration—US Public Health Service Health Evaluation and Enhancement Program. *American Journal of Cardiology*, **30**, 784-790.

Durnin, J.V.G.A. (1973). Nutrition. In J.C. Brocklehurst (Ed.), *Textbook of geriatric medicine and gerontology* (pp. 384-404). Edinburgh: Churchill-Livingstone.

Dwyer, J.F., & Bowes, M.D. (1979). Benefit-cost analysis for appraisal of recreation alternatives. *Journal of Forestry*, **77**(3).

Easterlin, R.A. (1978). What will 1984 be like? Socio-economic implications of recent twists in age structure. *Demography*, **15**, 397-432.

Eisdorfer, C. (1969). Intellectual and cognition changes in the aged. In E.W. Busse & E. Pfeiffer (Eds.), *Behaviour and adaptation in late life* (212-227). Boston: Little, Brown & Co.

Ellis, J.B. (1982). *Economic impacts of sport, recreation and fitness activities in Ontario: A preliminary review*. Ontario: Ontario Ministry of Tourism and Recreation.

Erikssen, J., Forfang, K., & Jervell, J. (1981). Coronary risk factors and physical fitness in healthy middle-aged men. *Acta Medica Scandinavica Supplement*, **645**, 57-64.

Erwin, J. (1978). People's Jewelry Company: Where a new personnel director introduced recreation and employee services and watched absenteeism fall dramatically. *Recreation Management*, **21**, 18-19.

Eskola, J., Runskanen, O., Soppi, E., Viljanen, M.K., Jarvinen, M., Toivonen, H., & Kouvalainen, K. (1978). Effect of sport stress on lymphocyte transformation and antibody formation. *Clinical and Experimental Immunology*, **32**, 339-345.

Espenschade, T.J., & Serow, W.J. (1978). *The economic consequences of slowing population growth*. New York: Academic Press.

Etzioni, A. (1978). Individual will and social conditions. *Annals of the American Academy of Political Social Science*, **437**, 62-73.

Fabun, D. (1971). *Dimensions of change*. Beverly Hills, CA: Glencoe Press.

Farrell, P.A., Gate, W.K., Maskeid, M.G., & Morgan, W.P. (1982). Increases in plasma ß-endorphin/ß-lipotropin immune reactivity after treadmill exercise in humans. *Journal of Applied Physiology*, **52**, 1245-1249.

Felton, J.S. (1971). Occupation. In L.A. Larson (Ed.), *Encyclopedia of sports sciences and medicine* (pp. 965-974). New York: MacMillan.

Fentem, P., & Bassey, E.J. (1977). *The case for exercise.* Working Paper #8. London: United Kingdom Sports Council.

Ferland, Y. (1980, November). Schooling and leisure activities. *Canadian Statistical Review,* vi-ix.

Fielding, J.E. (1982). Effectiveness of employee health improvement programs. *Journal of Occupational Medicine,* **24,** 907-916.

Finney, C. (1979). Recreation: Its effects on productivity. A recent study and its unexpected results. *Recreation Management,* **21,** 10.

Fishbein, M., & Ajzen, I. (1974). Attitudes towards objects as predictors of single and multiple behavioral criteria. *Psychological Review,* **81,** 59-74.

Fitch, E.M., & Shanklin, J.F. (1970). *The bureau of outdoor recreation.* New York: Praeger.

Fitness & Amateur Sport. (1983a). *Canadian youth and physical activity.* Ottawa: Fitness and Amateur Sport.

Fitness & Amateur Sport. (1983b). *Fitness and lifestyle in Canada.* Ottawa: Fitness and Amateur Sport.

Fitness Ontario. (1981). *Physical activity patterns in Ontario.* Toronto: Ministry of Culture and Recreation.

Flay, B.R., & Schlegel, R.P. (1980). *Mass media in health promotion: An analysis using an extended information-processing model.* Unpublished report, University of Waterloo.

Fletcher, C.M. (1959). Chronic bronchitis. Its prevalence, nature and pathogenesis. *American Review of Respiratory Disease,* **80,** 483-494.

Folkins, C.H. (1976). Effects of physical training on mood. *Journal of Clinical Psychology,* **32,** 385-388.

Foot, D.K. (1981). *A challenge of the 1980s. Unemployment and labour force growth in Canada and the provinces.* Toronto: Institute for Policy Analysis.

Foot, D.K. (1982). The economic impacts of aging in Canada. Macroeconomic indicators and policy implications. *Canadian Journal on Aging,* **1,** 60-71.

Fox, S., & Haskell, W.L. (1968). Physical activity and the prevention of coronary heart disease. *Bulletin of the New York Academy of Sciences,* **44,** 950-965.

Fraser, R.D. (1983). Funding and policy issues for the 80s and 90s. In B.P. Squires (Ed.), *Proceedings of the Conference on Health in the 80s and 90s and its impact on health sciences education* (pp. 149-171). Toronto: Council of Ontario Universities.

Friedman, E.A., & Havighurst, R.J. (1954). *The meaning of work and retirement.* Chicago: University of Chicago Press.

Friedman, M., & Rosenman, R.H. (1974). *Type A behaviour and your heart.* Greenwich, CT: Fawcett Crest Books.

Friedmann, E.A., & Orbach, H.L. (1974). Adjustment to retirement. In S. Arieti (Ed.), *American handbook of psychiatry I* (2nd ed., pp. 609-645). New York: Basic Books.

Fulgraff, B. (1971). Possible substitutes for work as the productive activity decreases (in the case of flexible retirement). In J. Huet (Ed.), *Work and aging.* Paris: International Centre of Social Gerontology.

Galevskaya, E.N. (1970). On the system and timing of gymnastic exercises for skilled industrial labourers at work. *Theory and Practice of Physical Culture* (Moscow), **7**, 52-54. [Cited by N. Schneidman. (1972, October). Soviet Studies in the fitness of the aged. *Canadian Family Physician*, 53-56.]

Gamble, H.B. (1975). Regional impacts from outdoor recreation. In B. Van der Smissen (Ed.), *Indicators of change in the recreation environment—A national research symposium* (pp. 1073-1078). University Park: Penn State University.

Garson, R.D. (1977). *Pilot project on Metropolitan Life Fitness program.* Unpublished report. Metropolitan Life Assurance Co.

Gary, V., & Guthrie, D. (1972). The effect of jogging on physical fitness and self concept in hospitalized alcoholics. *Quarterly Journal of Studies in Alcoholism*, **33**, 221-242.

Geiss, C.G., Hicks, W.W., & Londeree, B.R. (1978). Wage trends, recreation and national health. *Journal of Leisure Research*, **10**, 141-149.

Geissler, H.J. (1960). Zu einigen Untersuchungsergebnissen auf dem Gebiete der Ausgleichsgymnastik wahrend der Arbeitszeit. *Wissenschaft Zeitschrift Deutsches Hochschule Für Kultur* (Leipzig), **3**, 229-242.

Gibson, J.G. (1975). Problems of measuring recreation benefits with dual pricing systems. In G.A. Searle (Ed.), *Recreational economics and analyses* (pp. 36-52). Harlow, Essex: Longman.

Glenn, N.D., & Grimes, M. (1968). Aging, voting and political interest. *American Sociological Review*, **33**, 563-575.

Godin, G., & Shephard, R.J. (1983). Physical fitness promotion programmes: Effectiveness in modifying exercise behaviour. *Canadian Journal of Sport Sciences*, **8**, 104-113.

Godin, G., & Shephard, R.J. (1984). Physical fitness—Individual or societal responsibility? *Canadian Journal of Public Health*, **75**, 200-203.

Godin, G., & Shephard, R.J. (in press). Psychosocial factors influencing intentions to exercise of young students from grades 7 to 9. *Research Quarterly for Exercise and Sport*.

Gold, S. (1972). Non-use of neighbourhood parks. *Journal of American Institute of Planners*, **38**, 369-378.

Goldberg, H.M., Cohn, H.S., Dehn, T., & Seeds, R. (1980, June). Diagnosis and management of low back pain. *Occupational Health and Safety*, **49**, 14-15, 24-25.

Goodell, B.W. (1985). Death and dying. In R. Andres, E.L. Bierman, & W.R. Hazzard (Eds.), *Principles of geriatric medicine* (p. 960). New York: McGraw-Hill.

Gori, G.B., & Richter, B.J. (1978). Macro-economics of disease prevention in the United States. *Science*, **200**, 1124-1130.

Gray, J.A.M., Young, A., & Ennis, J.R. (1983). Promotion of exercise at work. *British Medical Journal*, **286**, 1958-1959.

Grayson, A.J., Sidaway, R.M., & Thompson, F.P. (1975). Some aspects of recreation planning in the forestry commission. In G.A. Searle (Ed.), *Recreational economics and analysis* (pp. 89-107). Harlow, Essex: Longman.

Greater London Council. (1976). *Greater London Recreation Study Part 3*. London: Greater London Council.

Green, L.W. (1979). How to evaluate health promotion. *Hospitals*, **53**, 106-108.

Green, L.W., Kreuter, M.W., Deeds, S.G., & Portridge, K.B. (1980). *Health education planning—A diagnostic approach*. Palo Alto, CA: Mayfield Publishing.

Groth-Junker, A.M. (1983, March 22). Home care for the elderly. *Medical Post*, p. 48.

Groves, D.L. (1980). A system-analysis of benefits from the industrial recreation environment. *Journal of Environmental Systems*, **10**, 1-16.

Groves, D.L., & DeCarlo, W.B. (1981). Job satisfaction and productivity and the role of employee recreation. *Recreation Management*, **24**, 29-30.

Guthrie, D.I. (1963). A new approach to handling in industry. A rational approach to the prevention of low back pain. *South African Medical Journal, 37*, 651-656.

Haggerty, R.J. (1977). Changing lifestyles to improve health. *Preventive Medicine, 6*, 276-289.

Hanke, H. (1979). *Freizeit in der DDR*. Berlin: Dietz Verlag.

Harris, C. (1983, March 12). Inflation takes a big toll over the decade. *Financial Post* (p. 10).

Haskell, W.L. (1978). Cardiovascular complications during exercise training of cardiac patients. *Circulation, 57*, 920-924.

Haskell, W.L., & Blair, S.N. (1980). The physical activity component of health promotion programs in occupational settings. *Public Health Reports, 95*, 109-118.

Hatry, H., & Dunn, D. (1971). *Measuring the effectiveness of local services: Recreation*. Washington, DC: The Urban Institute.

Heaps, R.A., & Thorstenson, C.T. (1974). Self-concept changes immediately and one year after survival training. *Therapeutic Recreation Journal, 8*, 60-63.

Hedfords, E., Holm, C., & Ohnell, B. (1976). Variations of blood lymphocytes during work studied by cell surface markers, DNA synthesis and cytotoxicity. *Clinical and Experimental Immunology, 24*, 328-335.

Heinzelmann, F. (1975). Psychosocial implications of physical activity. In S. Keir (Ed.), *Employee physical fitness in Canada* (pp. 33-43). Ottawa: Information Canada.

Heinzelmann, F., & Bagley, R. (1970). Response to physical activity programs and their effects on health behavior. *Public Health Reports, 85*, 905-911.

Henderson, J.M. (1974). The effect of physical conditioning on self-concept in college females. *Dissertation Abstracts International, 35*(6-B), 3063.

Henle, P. (1972, March). Recent growth of paid leisure for U.S. workers. *Monthly Labor Review*, p. 256.

Herzlich, C. (1973). *Health and illness*. London: Academic Press.

Hetherington, R.W., & Calderone, G.E. (1983). *Prevention and health policy: A view from the social sciences*. Rockville, MD: U.S. National Center for Health Services Research.

Hickey, N., Mulcahy, R., Bourke, G.J., Graham, I., & Wilson-Davis, K. (1975). Study of coronary risk factors related to physical activity in 15,171 men. *British Medical Journal, 3*, 507-509.

Hjelte, G., & Shivers, J.S. (1978). *Public administration of recreational services* (2nd ed.). Philadelphia: Lea & Febiger.

Hofstadter, R. (1955). *The age of reform.* New York: Vintage Books.

Holme, I., Helgeland, A., Hjermann, I., Leren, P., & Lund-Larsen, P.G. (1981). Physical activity at work and at leisure in relation to coronary risk factors and social class. A four year mortality follow up. The Oslo study. *Acta Medica Scandinavica,* **209,** 277-283.

Holmes, T.H., & Rahe, R.H. (1967). The social readjustment scale. *Journal of Psychosomatic Research,* **11,** 213-218.

Howard, J.H., Cunningham, D.A., & Rechnitzer, P.A. (1975). Health patterns associated with type A behaviour: A managerial population. *Working Paper Series, 145.* London, Ontario: University of Western Ontario, School of Business Administration.

Howard, J.H., Marshall, J., Rechnitzer, P.A., Cunningham, D.A., & Donner, A. (1982). Adapting to retirement. *Journal of the American Geriatric Society,* **30,** 488-500.

Howard, J.H., & Michalachki, A. (1979). Fitness and employee productivity. *Canadian Journal of Applied Sport Science,* **4,** 191-198.

Howell, M., & Howell, R. (1982). A model for national fitness programmes. *Proceedings of Sports Medicine Congress, Brisbane.* Melbourne: Australian Sports Medicine Federation.

Hudson, R.B., & Binstock, R.H. (1976). Political systems and aging. In R.H. Binstock & E. Shanas (Eds.), *Handbook of aging and the social sciences* (pp. 369-400). New York: Van Nostrand Reinhold.

Hughes, C.A. (1974). A comparison of the effects of four teaching techniques of body conditioning upon physical fitness and self concept. *Dissertation Abstracts International,* **34**(7A), 3857-3958.

Industrial Health Assistance Ltd. (1978). Unpublished research memo. Toronto.

Ingham, A., & Beamish, R. (1983). The maturation of industrial capitalism and the bourgeoisification of America's ludic interests. In E. Dunning (Ed.), *Sport and industrial change.* London: E. & F. Spon.

Innes, J.A., Campbell, I.W., Campbell, C.J., Needle, A.L., & Munroe, J.F. (1974). Long-term follow-up of therapeutic starvation. *British Medical Journal,* **2,** 357-359.

Isacsson, S.O. (1972). Venous occlusion plethysmography in 55 year old men. *Acta Medica Scandinavica Supplement,* **537,** 1-62.

Jacobs, P., & Chovil, A. (1983). Economic evaluation of corporate medical programs. *Journal of Occupational Medicine, 25,* 273-278.

Jenkins, A. (1974). *The case for squash: Its growth, development and prospects.* London Squash Rackets Association.

Jenkins, C., Bonser, K., Knapp, B., & Collins, M.F. (1981). *The impact of rugby sports centre* (Report to Sports Council by Department of Physical Education, Birmingham University). Birmingham, U.K.: Birmingham University.

Jensen, C.R. (1977). *Leisure and recreation: Introduction and overview.* Philadelphia: Lea & Febiger.

John Paul II. (1981). Papal Encyclical "On Human Work." Vatican City.

Jokl, E. (1931). Serologische untersuchungen an sportsleuten. *Zeitschrift für Experimentelle Medizin, 77,* 65-101.

Jokl, E. (1977). The immunological status of athletes. In D. Brunner & E. Jokl (Eds.), *The role of exercise in internal medicine.* Basel: S. Karger.

Kahn, H.A. (1963). The relationship of reported coronary heart disease mortality to physical activity of work. *American Journal of Public Health, 53,* 1058-1067.

Kannel, W.B. (1979). Some health benefits of physical activity. The Framingham Study. *Archives of Internal Medicine, 139,* 856-861.

Karson, S.G. (1982). A new emphasis on health promotion: The insurance business. *Health Education Quarterly, 9* (Suppl.), 42-48.

Kates, Peat, Marwick & Co. (1970). *Tourism and recreation in Ontario. Concepts of a system's model framework.* Toronto: Ministry of Tourism and Information.

Katz, S. (1980, September 27). The lost weekday. *Financial Post,* pp. 28-31.

Kavanagh, J.M., Marcus, M.J., & Gay, R.M. (1973). *Program budgeting for urban recreation. Current status and prospects in Los Angeles.* New York: Praeger.

Kavanagh, T., & Shephard, R.J. (1977). The effects of continued training on the aging process. *Annals of New York Academy of Sciences, 303,* 656-670.

Keelor, R. (1976, July 21). *Testimony to the U.S. Council on Wage and Price Stability Hearings on Health Care Costs.* Chicago.

King, B. (1981, September 19). Premium reward for kicking habit. *Financial Post,* p. 29.

Klarman, H.E. (1964). Socio-economic impact of heart disease. In E.C. Andrus (Ed.), *The heart and circulation. Vol. 2.* 2nd national conference on cardiovascular diseases. Community Services and Education. Washington, DC: U.S. Public Health Service.

Klarman, H.E. (1974). Application of cost-benefit analysis to health systems technology. *Journal of Occupational Medicine, 16,* 172-186.

Klarman, H.E. (1981). Economics of health. In D.W. Clark & B. MacMahon (Eds.), *Preventive and community medicine* (2nd ed., pp. 603-615). Boston: Little, Brown & Co.

Klempner, M.S., & Gallin, J.I. (1978). Inhibition of neutrophil Fc receptor function by corticosteroids. *Clinical and Experimental Immunology, 34,* 137-142.

Kmuzoz, Y.I. (1975). Role of physical culture in increasing labour productivity. *Yessis Review, 10*(3).

Knezevich, T. (1980). *Employee fitness motivation program pilot project results. October 1979-February 1980.* Ontario: Health Services Department, Health and Safety Division.

Kohn, R., & White, K.I. (1976). *Health care. An international study.* London: Oxford University Press.

Koplan, J.P., Powell, K.E., Sikes, R.K., Shirley, R.W., & Campbell, C.C. (1982). An epidemiological study of the benefits and risks of running. *Journal of the American Medical Association, 248,* 3118-3121.

Kowet, D. (1977). *The rich who own sports.* New York: Random House.

Kraus, R. (1971). *Recreation and leisure in modern society.* New York: Appleton Century Crofts.

Krause, B.L., Gibbs, D.R., & Brown, A.H. (1977, December 28). Is coronary artery surgery so expensive? *New Zealand Medical Journal, 86,* 570-572.

Kristein, M.M. (1977). Economic issues in prevention. *Preventive Medicine, 6,* 252-264.

Kristein, M.M. (1982). The economics of health promotion at the work site. *Health Education Quarterly, 9* (Suppl.), 27-36.

Kuhl, P.H., Koch-Nielsen, I., & Westergaard, K. (1966). *Fritidsvaner i Danmark.* Copenhagen: Teknisk Vorlag.

Kukkonen, K., Rauramaa, R., Siitonen, O., & Hänninen, O. (1982a). Physical training of obese middle-aged persons. *Annals of Clinical Research, 14* (Suppl. 34), 80-85.

Kukkonen, K., Rauramaa, R., Voutilainen, E., & Länsimies, E. (1982b). Physical training of middle-aged men with borderline hypertension. *Annals of Clinical Research*, **34**, 139-145.

Labonté, R., & Penfold, S. (1981). Canadian perspectives in health promotion: A critique. *Health Education*, **19**, 4-9.

LaFramboise, J.S. (1973). Health policy. Breaking it down into more manageable segments. *Canadian Medical Association Journal*, **108**, 388-393.

Lalonde, M. (1974). *A new perspective on the health of Canadians*. Ottawa: Information Canada.

Lalonde, M. (1978). Allocution, Ministre, Santé et bien-être social Canada. In F. Landry & W.A.R. Orban (Eds.), *Physical activity and human wellbeing* (pp. 9-105). Miami, FL: Symposia Specialists.

Landry, F., LeBlanc, C., Gaudreau, J., & Moisan, A. (1982). Fitness and health hazard indices: Observations on their relationships as discriminant criteria. *Canadian Journal of Public Health*, **73**, 57-62.

Laporte, W. (1966). The influence of a gymnastic pause upon recovery following post-office work. *Ergonomics*, **9**, 501-506.

Lawler/Dean Partnership. (1982). *Fitness Ontario: Media awareness study*. Toronto: Ministry of Culture & Recreation.

Layman, E.M. (1972). Exercise and mental health. In W.A.R. Orban (Ed.), *Proceedings of National Conferences on Fitness and Health*, **2**, 33-70. Ottawa: Queen's Printer.

Layman, E.M. (1974). Psychological effects of physical activity. In J.H. Wilmore (Ed.), *Exercise and sports science reviews*. New York: Academic Press.

Leonardson, G., & Gargiulo, R.M. (1978). Self perception and physical fitness. *Perceptual and Motor Skills*, **46**, 338.

Levasseur, R., & Bellefleur, M. (1976). *Loisir Québec*. Montréal: Editions Bellarmin.

Lick, F.A. (1975). *Factors relating to use and non-use of neighbourhood parks in San Jose, California*. Unpublished master's thesis. San Jose State University.

Lindén, V. (1969). Absence from work and physical fitness. *British Journal of Industrial Medicine*, **26**, 47-53.

Lion, S. (1978). Psychological effects of jogging: A preliminary study. *Perceptual and Motor Skills*, **47**, 1215-1218.

Lipman, A. (1979). Impact of demographic changes on family. In H. Orimo, K. Shimada, M. Iriki, & D. Maeda (Eds.), *Recent advances in gerontology* (pp. 306-307). Amsterdam: Excerpta Medica.

Love, S. (1973, October/November). Venture or adventure? *Business Forum* (San Diego), **11**, 21.

Luce, B.R., & Schweitzer, S.O. (1978). Smoking and alcohol abuse: A comparison of their economic consequences. *New England Journal of Medicine*, **298**, 569-571.

Maccoby, N., & Farquhar, J.W. (1975). Communication for health: Unselling heart disease. *Journal of Community Health*, **25**, 114-126.

MacIntosh, D.L., Skrien, T., & Shephard, R.J. (1972). Physical activity and injury. A study of sports injuries at the University of Toronto, 1951-1968. *Journal of Sports Medicine and Physical Fitness*, **12**, 224-237.

MacLean-Hunter Research Bureau. (1977). *Canada's leisure market*. Toronto: MacLean-Hunter.

Manguroff, J., Channe, N., & Georgieff, N. (1960). Tempo, Dosierung, Anzahl und Charakter der Ubungen für Berufsgymnastik. Vuprosi na Fiz. Kult. *Sofia*, **5**, 161. [Quoted by Laporte (1966)]

Mansfield, N.L. (1971). The estimation of benefits from recreation sites and the provision of a new recreation facility. *Journal of Regional Studies*, **5**, 55-69.

Manuso, J.S.J. (1983). The Equitable Life Assurance Society Program. *Preventive Medicine*, **12**, 658-662.

Marans, R.W., & Fly, J.M. (1981). *Recreation and the quality of urban life*. Ann Arbor, MI: University of Michigan. Institute for Social Research.

Marsden, V. (1979). Fitness programming possibilities and considerations. In R. Wanzel (Ed.), *Employee fitness. The how to . . .* (pp. 55-68). Toronto: Ministry of Culture and Recreation.

Marsden, V., & Youlden, P. (1979, May). *Report to health & welfare committee on employee fitness programme*. Ottawa: Health & Welfare Canada.

Martin, J. (1978). Corporate health: A result of employee fitness. *The Physician and Sportsmedicine*, **6**, 135-137.

Martin, W.H., & Mason, S. (1979). *Broad patterns of leisure expenditure*. London: A state of the art review prepared for the Sports Council and Social Science Research Council joint panel on Leisure and Recreation Research. London: U.K. Sports Council.

Massie, J.F., & Shephard, R.J. (1971). Physiological and psychological effects of training. *Medicine and Science in Sports*, **3**, 110-117.

Matracia, S., & Matracia, R. (1980). Syndrome by fatigue in football-players. Immunologic modifications. In L. Vecchiet (Ed.), *1st International Congress on sports medicine applied to football* (pp. 51-64). Rome: D. Guanella.

Mazza, L. (1980). Immunological characteristics of the athlete. In L. Vecchiet (Ed.), *1st International Congress on sports medicine applied to football* (pp. 306-314).

McGinnis, J.M. (1981). Analyzing the moral issues in health promotion. *Preventive Medicine, 10,* 379-381.

McGinnis, J.M. (1982). Future directions in health promotion. In R.B. Taylor, J.R. Ureda, & J.W. Denham (Eds.), *Health promotion: Principles and clinical applications* (ch. 17). Englewood Cliffs, NJ: Prentice Hall.

McPherson, B.D. (1975). Sport consumption and the economics of consumerism. In D.W. Ball & J.W. Loy (Eds.), *Sport and social order—Contributions to the sociology of sport* (pp. 243-275). Reading, MA: Addison Wesley.

McPherson, B.D., & Kozlik, C.A. (1980). Canadian leisure patterns by age. Disengagement, continuity or ageism. In V.W. Marshall (Ed.), *Aging in Canada. Social perspectives* (pp. 113-122). Toronto: Fitzhenry & Whiteside.

Mealey, M. (1979). New fitness for police and firefighters. *The Physician and Sports Medicine, 7,* 96-100.

Medalie, J.H., Tyroler, H.A., & Heiss, G. (1980). High density lipoprotein cholesterol and ischemic heart disease. In C. Long (Ed.), *Prevention and rehabilitation in ischemic heart disease* (pp. 18-47). Baltimore: Williams & Wilkins.

Megalli, B. (1978, May). Employee fitness program: Philanthropic venture or shrewd investment. *Labour Gazette,* pp. 174-182.

Merrill Lynch. (1968). *Leisure investment opportunity in a $150 billion market.* New York: Securities Division, Merrill, Lynch, Pierce, Fenner & Smith.

Merwin, D.J., & Northrop, B.A. (1982). Health action in the workplace: Complex issues—No simple answers. *Health Education Quarterly, 9* (Suppl.), 73-82.

Métivier, G. (1975). Elementary physical education: A sound investment for Canada's economy. *CAHPER Journal, 41,* 3-5.

Meyer, H.D., & Brightbill, C.K. (1964). *Community recreation: A guide to its organization.* Englewood Cliffs, NJ: Prentice Hall.

Michael, E.D. (1957). Stress adaptation through exercise. *Research Quarterly*, **28**, 50-54.

Miller, S.J. (1965). The social dilemma of the aging leisure participant. In A.M. Rose & W.A. Peterson (Eds.), *Older people and their social world*. Philadelphia: F.A. Davis.

Ministry of Education, Science and Culture. (1981). *Physical education and sports in Japan* (p. 14). Tokyo: Physical Education Bureau of Ministry of Education, Science & Culture.

Mishan, E.J. (1976). *Cost-benefit analysis*. New York: Praeger Publishing.

Montgomery, D.G. (1978). *Productivity, the older worker and recurrent education* (Abstract). 11th International Congress of Gerontology, Tokyo.

Mooney, G.H. (1977). *The valuation of human life*. London: MacMillan.

Morey, R.C. (1983). Cost-effectiveness of an employer-sponsored recreational program: A case study. *Omega*, **14**, 67-74.

Morgan, P., Gildiner, M., & Wright, G.R. (1976, May/June). Smoking reduction in adults who take up exercise: A survey of running clubs for adults. *CAHPER Journal*, **42**, 39-43.

Morgan, R. (1977). *Prospects for preventive medicine*. A catalogue. Toronto: Ontario Economic Council.

Morgan, W.P., & Horstman, D.H. (1976). Anxiety reduction following acute physical activity. *Medicine and Science in Sports*, **8**, 62.

Morikawa, S. (1979). Fundamental problems in studies on amateur sport. Introduction to theories on "Sport Labour." *International Review of Sport Sociology*, **1**(14), 21-50.

Morris, J.N., Adams, C., Chave, S.P.N., Sirey, C., Epstein, L., & Sheehan, D.J. (1973). Vigorous exercise in leisure time and the incidence of coronary heart disease. *Lancet*, **(i)**, 333-339.

Morris, J.N., Heady, J.A., Raffle, P.A., Roberts, C.G., & Parks, J.W. (1953). Coronary heart disease and physical activity of work. *Lancet*, **(ii)**, 1053-1057, 1111-1120.

Muir-Gray, J.A. (1979). Choosing priorities. *Journal of Medical Ethics*, **5**, 73-75.

Mullen, P.D. (1981). Children as a national priority: Closing the gap between knowledge and policy. *Health Education Quarterly*, **8**, 15-24.

Murayama, S. (1979). Contribution of retired persons to society—Situation in Japan. In H. Orimo, K. Shimada, M. Iriki, & D. Maeda (Eds.), *Recent advances in gerontology* (pp. 381-382). Amsterdam: Excerpta Medica.

Murphy, J.F., Williams, J.G., Niepoth, E.W., & Brown, P.D. (1973). *Leisure service delivery system: A modern perspective*. Philadelphia: Lea & Febiger.

Nash, J.B. (1960). Philosophy of recreation and leisure. Dubuque, IA: W.C. Brown.

National Health & Welfare. (1980). *Health Information Division, Information Systems Directorate*. Policy Planning and Information Branch. Ottawa: National Health and Welfare.

Nescrow, H.L., Pompel, D.T., & Reich, C.M. (1975). Benefit-cost evaluation. *Parks and Recreation*, **10**, 29-30, 40.

Netherlands Sports Federation. (1980). *500 Sports Halls in Netherlands*. The Hague: Author.

Nienaber, J., & Wildavsky, A. (1973). *The budgeting and evaluation of federal recreation programs*. New York: Basic Books.

Nojima, M. (1978). Characteristics of leisure activities of the elderly. *Proceedings of 11th International Congress of Gerontology* (p. 207). Tokyo: Science and Medical Publications.

Noll, R.G. (1974). *Government and the sports business*. Washington, DC: Brookings Institute.

NorthWest Council for Sport and Recreation, United Kingdom. (1982). *The impact of a new sports centre on sports participation and sporting facilities*. A case study of the Atherton area 1976-1981. Manchester: Author.

Novelli, W.D., & Ziska, D. (1982). Health promotion in the workplace: An overview. *Health Education Quarterly*, **9** (Supplement), 20-26.

O'Hara, W., Allen, C., Shephard, R.J., & Allen, G. (1979). Fat loss in the cold: A controlled study. *Journal of Applied Physiology*, **46**, 872-877.

Oldridge, N.B. (1979). Compliance of post-myocardial infarction patients to exercise programs. *Medicine and Science in Sports*, **11**, 373-375.

Olsen, E. (1983, March). The cost of running. *Runner*.

Olson, J.M., & Zanna, M.P. (1981). *Promoting physical activity—A social psychological perspective*. Ontario: Ministry of Culture & Recreation.

Ontario civil servants' 1980 sick leaves cost $48 million. (1981, September 28). *Ottawa Citizen*.

Ontario Ministry of Tourism and Recreation. (1982, November). *Canadian Gallup Poll—Ontario Omnibus Survey*. Toronto, Ontario: Author.

Ontario Ministry of Tourism and Recreation. (1983). *Physical activity patterns in Ontario II*. Toronto: Author.

Orban, W.A.R. (1974). *Proceedings of the National Conference on Fitness and Health*. Ottawa: Health & Welfare, Canada.

Paffenbarger, R. (1977). Physical activity and fatal heart attack: Protection or selection? In E.A. Amsterdam, J.H. Wilmore, & A.N. de Maria (Eds.), *Exercise in cardiovascular health and disease* (pp. 35-49). New York: Yorke Medical Books.

Paffenbarger, R., Wing, A.L., & Hyde, R.T. (1978). Physical activity as an index of heart attack risk in college alumni. *American Journal of Epidemiology, 108*, 161-175.

Pafnote, M., Voida, I., & Luchian, O. (1979). Physical fitness in different groups of industrial workers. *Physiologie, 16*, 129-131.

Paillat, P. (1971). The cost of the advancement of retirement age in industrialized countries. In 2nd International Course in Social Gerontology, *Work and aging* (pp. 39-54). Paris: International Centre of Social Gerontology.

Paillat, P. (1977). *Implications for social security of research on aging and retirement* (pp. 4-20). Geneva: International Social Security Association.

Paillat, P. (1979). Retired people could help. In H. Orimo, K. Shimada, M. Iriki, & D. Maeda (Eds.), *Recent advances in gerontology* (pp. 383-384). Amsterdam: Excerpta Medica.

Palmore, E. (1970). Health practices and illness among the aged. *Gerontologist, 10*, 313-316.

Parker, S. (1971). *The future of work and leisure*. New York: Praeger.

Parker, S.R., Thomas, C.G., Ellis, N.D., & McCarthy, W.E.T. (1971). *Effects of the redundancy payments act*. London: Her Majesty's Stationery Office.

Parr, R.B., & Kerr, J.D. (1975). Liability and insurance. In P.K. Wilson (Ed.), *Adult fitness and cardiac rehabilitation* (pp. 219-224). Baltimore Park, MD: University Park Press.

Pate, R.R., & Blair, S.N. (1983). Physical fitness programming for health promotion at the worksite. *Preventive Medicine, 12*, 632-643.

Pauly, J.T., Palmer, J.A., Wright, C.C., & Pfeiffer, G.J. (1982). The effect of a 14-week employee fitness program on selected physiological and psychological parameters. *Journal of Occupational Medicine, 24*, 457-463.

Pearson, N. (1969). *Planning for a leisure society*. Guelph, Ontario: Centre for Resources Development.

Peepre, M. (1978). *Employee fitness and lifestyle project*. Ottawa: Fitness and Amateur Sport Directorate, Health and Welfare, Canada.

Pellegrino, E.D. (1981). Health promotion as public policy: The need for moral groundings. *Preventive Medicine,* **10**, 371-378.

Peters, K.R., Benson, H., & Porter, D. (1977). Daily relaxation response breaks in a working population: Effects on self-reported measures of health, performance, and well-being. *American Journal of Public Health,* **67**, 946-952.

Plato. (1937). *The dialogues of Plato* (p. 143, B. Jowett, Trans.). New York: Random House.

Plutchik, R., Conte, H., & Weiner, M.B. (1973). Studies on body image II. Dollar values of body parts. *Journal of Gerontology,* **28**, 89-91.

Pollock, M. (1973). The quantification of endurance training. *Exercise and Sport Science Reviews,* **1**, 155-188.

Powell, B.J., & Martin, J.K. (1980). Economic implications of Canada's aging society. In V. Marshall (Ed.), *Aging and society* (pp. 204-214). Toronto: Fitzhenry & Whiteside.

Pratt, H.J. (1976). *The gray lobby.* Chicago: University of Chicago Press.

Pravosudov, V.P. (1978). Effects of physical exercises on health and economic efficiency. In F. Landry & W.A.R. Orban (Eds.), *Physical activity and human well-being* (pp. 261-271). Miami, FL: Symposia Specialists.

President's Council on Physical Fitness and Sports. (1973, May). *Newsletter—Special edition.* Washington, DC: Author.

Pyfer, H.R., & Doane, B.L. (1973). Aspects of community exercise programs. Economic aspects of cardiac rehabilitation programs. In J.P. Naughton, H.K. Hellerstein, & I.C. Mohler (Eds.), *Exercise testing and exercise training in coronary heart disease* (pp. 365-369). New York: Academic Press.

Pyle, R.L. (1979). Performance measures for corporate fitness programs. *Human Resources Management,* **18**(3).

Quasar. (1976). *The relationships between physical fitness and the cost of health care.* Toronto: Quasar Systems Ltd.

Raab, W., & Gilman, S.B. (1964). Insurance sponsored preventative cardiac reconditioning centers in West Germany. *American Journal of Cardiology,* **13**, 670-673.

Redlich, F. (1965). Leisure-time activities. A historical, sociological and economic analysis. *Explorations in Entrepreneurial History,* **3**, 3-23.

Reed, J.D. (1981, November 2). America shapes up. *Time*, pp. 64-79.

Réville, P.H. (1970). *Sport for all. Physical activity and the prevention of disease*. Strasbourg: Council of Europe.

Rhodes, A. (1982, May). Don't weight for summer. *Financial Post Magazine*, pp. 83-84.

Rice, D.P. (1966). *Estimating the cost of illness*. Washington, DC: U.S. Government Printing Office.

Richardson, B. (1974, May/June). Don't just sit there—Exercise something. *Fitness for Living*, **49**.

Richardson, I.M. (1964). *Age and need: A study of older people in North-East Scotland*. London: Livingstone.

Rickey, C.W. (1972). Value and property taxes of a seasonal home subdivision. Case study. *Land Economics*, **48**, 387-392.

Riley, M.W., Johnson, M.E., & Foner, A. (1972). *Aging and society: Vol. 3. A sociology of stratification*. New York: Russell Sage Foundation.

Ritchie, J.R.B. (1974). Leisure: An economic or social phenomenon. *Optimum*, **5**, 40-51.

Roberts, A.D. (1982). *The economic benefits of participation in regular physical activity*. Canberra, Australia: Recreation Ministers' Council of Australia.

Roberts, C., & Wall, G. (1979). Possible impacts of Vaughan Theme Park. *Recreation Research Review*, **7**, 11-14.

Roberts, J. (1979). *The commercial sector in leisure*. London: United Kingdom Sports Council.

Roberts, J., & Maurer, K. (1977). *Blood pressure levels of persons 6-74 years, U.S. 1971-74*. National Center for Health Statistics. (DHEW Publication No. HRA 78-1648). Washington, DC: U.S. Government Printing Office.

Roccella, E.J. (1982). Selected roles of the federal government and health promotion/disease prevention—Focus on the worksetting. *Health Education Quarterly*, **9** (Suppl.), 83-91.

Rochmis, P., & Blackburn, H. (1971). Exercise tests. A survey of procedures, safety and litigation experience in approximately 170,000 tests. *Journal of the American Medical Association*, **217**, 1061-1066.

Rodale, R. (1983). The Rodale press program. *Preventive Medicine*, **12**, 663-666.

Rodgers, B. (1978). *Rationalising sports policies—Sport in its social context. International Comparisons, Technical Supplement*. Strasbourg: Committee for the Development of Sport—Council of Europe.

Rogers, P.J., Eaton, E.K., & Bruhn, J.G. (1981). Is health promotion cost effective? *Preventive Medicine*, **10**, 324-339.

Rogot, E., & Murray, J.L. (1980). Smoking and causes of death among U.S. veterans: 16 years of observation. *Public Health Reports*, **95**, 213-222.

Rohmert, W. (1973). Problems in determining rest allowances. Part I. Use of modern methods to evaluate stress and strain in static muscular work. *Applied Ergonomics*, **4**, 91-95.

Rose, G. (1970). Changing incidence of disease. In R.J. Jones (Ed.), *Atherosclerosis: Proceedings of the Second International Symposium* (pp. 310-314). New York: Springer.

Rosow, J.M. (1977). Self-managed teams at Butler plant, cuts costs, raises profitability. *World of Work Report*, **2**, 124-125.

Ross, D.N. (1978). *Economics of chronic disability and frailty in old age: Lessons from the comparative cost of various forms of institutional and day care* (Abstracts). 11th International Congress of Gerontology, Tokyo.

Sachs, M.L. (1982). Compliance and addiction to exercise. In R.C. Cantu (Ed.), *The exercising adult* (pp. 19-27). Lexington, MA: D.C. Heath.

Sackett, D.L., Chambers, L.W., MacPherson, A.S., Goldsmith, C.H., & McAuley, R.G. (1977). The development and application of indices of health: General methods and a summary of results. *American Journal of Public Health*, **67**, 423-428.

Santa Barbara, J. (1982a). *Evaluation of the Thunder Bay community fitness campaign*. Ontario: Ministry of Culture and Recreation.

Santa Barbara, J. (1982b). *The relationship between physical activity and other health-related lifestyle behaviours*. Toronto: Ontario Ministry of Tourism and Recreation.

Sauvy, A. (1970). Demographic and economic aspects of the retirement problem. In J.A. Huet (Ed.), *1st International course in social gerontology* (pp. 15-36). Paris: International Centre of Social Gerontology.

Sawyer, J.A. (1979). Prospects and policies for economic growth. *Economic Policy Review*, **1**, 11-25.

Schelling, T.C. (1968). The life you save may be your own. In S.B. Chase (Ed.), *Problems in public expenditure* (pp. 127-162). Washington, DC: Brookings Institution.

Schrank, H.T., & Riley, J.W. (1978). *Retirees who don't retire: Their contribution to work groups* (Abstracts). 11th International Congress of Gerontology, Tokyo.

Schutjer, W.A., & Hallberg, M.C. (1968). Impact of water recreational development on rural property values. *American Journal of Agricultural Economics, 50*, 572-583.

Schwenger, C.W. (1976). *Future needs in retirement.* [National nutrition seminar]. Toronto: General Foods.

Schwenger, C.W., & Gross, M.J. (1980). Institutional care and institutionalization of the elderly in Canada. In V.W. Marshall (Ed.), *Aging in Canada* (pp. 248-256). Toronto: Fitzhenry & Whiteside.

Scottish Sports Council. (1980). *A question of balance.* Edinburgh: Scottish Sports Council.

Segall, A. (1981). Socio-cultural variation in sick role behavioural expectations. In D. Coburn, C. D'Arcy, P. New, & G. Torrance (Eds.), *Health and Canadian society* (pp. 171-179). Toronto: Fitzhenry & Whiteside.

Selye, H. (1974). Stress and the nation's health. In *Proceedings of the National Conference on Fitness and Health* (pp. 65-74). Ottawa: Health and Welfare, Canada.

Shain, M., & Groeneveld, J. (1980). *Employee assistance programs: Philosophy, theory and practice.* Toronto: Lexington Books.

Shanas, E. (1971). Disengagement and work: Myth and reality. In J.A. Huet (Ed.), *Work and aging.* Paris: International Centre of Social Gerontology.

Shapiro, S., Weinblatt, E., Frank, C.W., & Sager, R.V. (1969). Incidence of coronary heart disease in a population insured for medical care (H.I.P.). *American Journal of Public Health, 59* (Suppl. 2), 1-101.

Shaver, L.A., & Tobin, S. (1978). *Propensity to retire when income fear is reduced* (Abstracts). 11th International Congress of Gerontology, Tokyo.

Schechter, M., & Lucas, R.C. (1978). *Simulation of recreational use for park and wilderness management.* Baltimore: Johns Hopkins Press.

Shephard, R.J. (1974). *Men at work: Application of ergonomics to performance and design.* Springfield, IL: C.C. Thomas.

Shephard, R.J. (1975). Future research on the quantifying of endurance training. *Journal of Human Ergology, 3*, 163-181.

Shephard, R.J. (1977a). Coronary artery disease—The magnitude of the problem. In T. Kavanagh (Ed.), *International Symposium on Exercise and Coronary Artery Disease* (pp. 1-16). Toronto: Toronto Rehabilitation Centre.

Shephard, R.J. (1977b). *Endurance fitness* (2nd ed.). Toronto: University of Toronto Press.

Shephard, R.J. (1978). *Physical activity and aging*. London: Croom Helm.

Shephard, R.J. (1979). Current status of the Canadian Home Fitness Test. *South African Journal for Research in Sport, Physical Education and Recreation, 2*, 19-35.

Shephard, R.J. (1981). *Ischemic heart disease and physical activity*. Chicago: Year Book Publishers.

Shephard, R.J. (1982a). *Physical activity and growth*. Chicago: Year Book Publishers.

Shephard, R.J. (1982b). Prognostic value of exercise testing for ischaemic heart disease. *British Journal of Sports Medicine, 16*, 220-229.

Shephard, R.J. (1983a). Can we identify those for whom exercise is hazardous? *Sports Medicine* (Auckland), *1*, 75-86.

Shephard, R.J. (1983b). Economics of the fitness industries—The Canadian scene since 1966. *Journal of Sports Medicine and Physical Fitness, 22*, 245-258.

Shephard R.J. (1983c). Exercise and the healthy mind. *Canadian Medical Association Journal, 128*, 525-530.

Shephard, R.J. (1984). *Fitness and health in industry*. Springfield, IL: C.C. Thomas.

Shephard, R.J., Corey, P., & Cox, M. (1982). Health hazard appraisal—The influence of an employee fitness programme. *Canadian Journal of Public Health, 73*, 183-187.

Shephard, R.J., Corey, P., Renzland, P., & Cox, M.H. (1982). The influence of an industrial fitness programme upon medical care costs. *Canadian Journal of Public Health, 73*(4), 259-263.

Shephard, R.J., Corey, P., Renzland, P., & Cox, M. (1983). The impact of changes in fitness and lifestyle upon health care utilization. *Canadian Journal of Public Health, 74*, 51-54.

Shephard, R.J., Cox, M., & Corey, P. (1981). Fitness program participation: Its effects on worker performance. *Journal of Occupational Medicine, 23*, 359-363.

Shephard, R.J., Kavanagh, T., Tuck, J., & Kennedy, J. (1983). Marathon jogging in post-myocardial infarction patients. *Journal of Cardiac Rehabilitation, 3*, 321-329.

Shephard, R.J., & LaBarre, R. (1976). *Attitudes to smoking and cigarette smoke. The Toronto Survey.* Willowdale, Ontario: York-Toronto Respiratory Disease Association.

Shephard, R.J., & LaBarre, R. (1978). Current attitudes towards smoking in Toronto. *Canadian Journal of Public Health, 69*(2), 121-126.

Shephard, R.J., Morgan, P., Finucane, R., & Schimmelfing, L. (1980). Factors influencing recruitment to an occupational fitness program. *Journal of Occupational Medicine, 22*, 389-398.

Sheppard, H. (1971). The importance of the older worker in the economy of the nation (2). In J.A. Huet (Ed.), *Work and aging* (pp. 31-38). Paris: Centre of Social Gerontology.

Sidney, K.H. (1975). *Responses of elderly subjects to a program of progressive exercise training.* Unpublished doctoral dissertation, University of Toronto, Toronto, Ontario.

Sidney, K.H., & Shephard, R.J. (1976). Attitudes towards health and physical training in the elderly. Effects of a physical training program. *Medicine and Science in Sports, 8*, 246-252.

Sidney, K.H., Shephard, R.J., & Harrison, J. (1977). Endurance training and body composition of the elderly. *American Journal of Clinical Nutrition, 30*, 326-333.

Sielaff, R.O. (1964). *The economics of outdoor recreation in the upper mid-west.* Duluth, MN: Social Sciences Research Foundation.

Simanis, J.G., & Coleman, J.R. (1980). Health care expenditures in nine industrialized countries, 1960-76. *Social Security Bulletin, 43*, 3-8.

Singer Associates. (1982). Comments on the Economic Statement by the Honourable Marc Lalonde, Minister of Finance. *Canadian Quarterly Economics Review*, Special Issue.

Slee, D., & Peepre, M. (1974, May). *Report to Health and Welfare Committee on employee fitness programme.* Ottawa: Health and Welfare Canada.

Sloan, A.W., Koeslag, J.H., & Bredell, G.A. (1973). Body composition, work capacity and work efficiency of active and inactive young men. *European Journal of Applied Physiology, 32*, 17-24.

Smith, C.R., Partain, L.E., & Champlin, J.R. (1966). *Rural recreation for profit.* Danville, IL: Interstate Printers and Publishers.

Smith, E.L., & Babcock, S.W. (1973). Effects of physical activity on bone loss in the aged. *Medicine and Science in Sports*, **5**, 68.

Smith, P.C., Kendal, L.M., & Hulin, C.L. (1969). *The measurement of satisfaction in work and retirement*. Chicago: Rand McNally.

Smith, R.J. (1975). Problems of interpreting recreation benefits from a recreation demand curve. In G.A. Searle (Ed.), *Recreational economics and analysis* (pp. 62-74). Harlow, Essex: Longman.

Smith, S.L.J. (1983). *Recreation geography*. Harlow, Essex: Longman.

Smith, V.K., & Krutilla, J.V. (1976). *Structure and properties of a wilderness travel simulator*. Baltimore: Johns Hopkins Press.

Song, T.K., Shephard, R.J., & Cox, M. (1982). Absenteeism, employee turnover and sustained exercise participation. *Journal of Sports Medicine and Physical Fitness*, **22**, 392-399.

Sorensen, C.H., & Sonne-Holm, S. (1981). Social costs of sports injuries. *British Journal of Sports Medicine*, **14**, 24-25.

Spode, H. (1980). Der deutsche Arbeiter Reist. Massentourismus in Dritten Reich. In G. Huck (Ed.), *Sozialgeschichte der Freizeit* (pp. 281-306). Wuppertal: Peter Hammer.

Sports Council. (1976). *Provision for playing pitches*. London: Sports Council.

Squires, B.P. (Ed.). (1982). *Conference on health in the 80s and 90s and its impact on health sciences education*. Toronto: Council of Ontario Universities.

Stallings, W.M., O'Rourke, T.W., & Gross, D. (1975). Professorial correlates of physical exercise. *Journal of Sports Medicine and Physical Fitness*, **15**, 333-336.

Statistics Canada. (1975). *Travel, tourism and outdoor recreation 1973/74*. (Catalogue CS 66-202/1974). Ottawa: Author.

Statistics Canada. (1976). *Culture statistics—Recreational activities*. (Occasional paper 87-501, pp. 1-94). Ottawa: Author.

Statistics Canada. (1979a). *Population projection for Canada and the provinces, 1976-2001*. (Catalogue 91-520 Occasional). Ottawa: Information Canada.

Statistics Canada. (1979b). *Travel, tourism and outdoor recreation: A statistical digest 1973 and 1974*. Ottawa: Author.

Statistics Canada. (1980). *Family expenditures in Canada*. (Occasional paper 62-550). Ottawa: Author.

Statistics Canada. (1981). *Travel, tourism and outdoor recreation—A statistical digest 1978 and 1979*. (Occasional paper 87-401). Ottawa: Author.

Steel, C.M., Evans, J., & Smith, M.A. (1974). Physiological variation in circulating B cell:T cell ratio in man. *Nature, 247*, 387-389.

Streib, G.F., & Streib, R.B. (1979). Retired persons and their contributions: Exchange theory. In H. Orimo, K. Shimada, M. Iriki, & D. Maeda (Eds.), *Recent advances in gerontology* (pp. 385-386). Amsterdam: Excerpta Medica.

Stundl, H. (1977). *Freizeit und Erholungsport in der DDR*. Schorndorf: Karl Hofmann.

Sue, R. (1982). *Vers une societé du temps libre*. Paris: Presses Universitaires de France.

Sugden, W.A. (1978). *The principles of practical cost-benefit analysis*. Oxford, England: Oxford University Press.

Süominen, H., Heikkinen, E., Parkatte, T., Forsberg, S., & Kiiskinen, A. (1977). Effects of "lifelong" physical training on functional aging in men. *Scandinavian Journal of Social Medicine Supplement, 14*, 225-240.

Superko, H.R., Bernauer, E., & Voss, J. (1983). Effects of a mandatory job performance test and voluntary remediation program on law enforcement personnel. *Medicine and Science in Sports and Exercise, 15*, 149-150.

System Three (Communications) Ltd. Sponsorship. (1973). *Commercial sponsorship of sport and other activities in the U.K.* London: Author.

Taylor, C. (1978). The activity park: Making small outdoor areas useful for fitness and hypaethral appreciation of older people. In *Proceedings of the 11th International Gerontological Congress* (p. 208). Tokyo: Science and Medicine Publications.

Taylor, H.L., Parkin, R.W., Blackburn, H., & Keys, A. (1966). Problems in the analysis of the relationship of coronary heart disease to physical activity or its lack, with special reference to sample size and occupational withdrawal. In K. Evang & K.L. Andersen (Eds.), *Physical activity in health and disease*. Baltimore: Williams & Wilkins.

Thomas, G.S. (1979). Physical activity and health: Epidemiologic and policy implications. *Preventive Medicine, 8*, 89-103.

Thompson, P.D., Funk, E.J., Carleton, R.A., & Sturner, W.Q. (1982). Sudden death during jogging: A study of the Rhode Island population from 1975 through 1980. *Medicine and Science in Sports and Exercise, 14*, 115.

Thorndike, A. (1942). *Athletic injuries. Prevention, diagnosis and treatment*. Philadelphia: Lea & Febiger.

Thornton, A.W. (1974). Mass communications and dental health behavior. *Health Education Monograph*, **2**, 201-208.

Thurow, L.C. (1980). *The zero-sum society*. New York: Basic Books.

Timiras, P.S. (1972). *Developmental physiology and aging*. New York: Macmillan.

Tindale, J.A., & Marshall, V.W. (1980). A generational-conflict perspective for gerontology. In V. Marshall (Ed.), *Aging in Canada* (pp. 43-50). Toronto: Fitzhenry & Whiteside.

Tobacco Tax Council. (1980). *The tax burden on tobacco: Historical compilation*. Richmond, VA: Author.

Toplin, H., & Bentkover, J.D. (1980). The economics of sports injuries. *Athletic Purchasing & Facilities*, **4**(9).

Torrance, G.W. (1976). Social preferences for health states: An empirical evaluation of three measurement techniques. *Socio-Economic Planning Sciences*, **10**, 129-136.

Tremblay, J.P. (1976). *Vienne le temps du loisir*. Montreal: Editions Pauline.

Tsalikis, G. (1980). Remodelling the staff of Aesculapius. *Social Science in Medicine*, **14A**, 97-106.

United Kingdom Sports Council. (1982a). *A forward look*. London: Sports Council.

United Kingdom Sports Council. (1982b). *Sports in the community: The next 10 years*. London: Sports Council.

U.S. Bureau of Outdoor Recreation. (1972). *Recreation land price escalation* (pp. 10-11). Washington, DC: Author.

U.S. Congress, Office of Technology Assessment. (1980). *The implications of cost-effectiveness analysis of medical technology: Background paper #1—Methodological issues and literature review*. Washington, DC: Author. [Cited by Drummond & Mooney, p. 1561]

U.S. Department of Commerce. (1964). *Tourist and recreation potential—Lafayette and Suwannee counties. Suwannee river area, Florida*. Washington, DC: Author.

U.S. Department of Commerce. (1977). *Bureau of the Census—U.S. county business patterns*. Washington, DC: U.S. Government Printing Office.

U.S. Department of Commerce. (1979). *Growth of selected leisure industries*. (Leisure services location package 79-22715, Item 582-E). Washington, DC: Author.

U.S. National Safety Council. (1943, October). Injuries from company-sponsored recreational activities. *National Safety Council Newsletter*, p. 10.

U.S. National Safety Council. (1980). *Accident Facts*. Chicago: Author.

U.S. Surgeon General. (1979). Healthy people. [The Surgeon General's Report on Health Promotion and Disease Prevention. DHEW Publication PHS/79/55071] Washington, DC: U.S. Government Printing Office.

Vander, L., Franklin, B.A., & Rubenfire, M. (1982). Cardiovascular complications of recreational physical activity: A retrospective survey. *Medicine and Science in Sports*, **14**, 115.

Veal, A.J. (1982). *Using sports centres*. London: The Sports Council.

Veatch, R.M. (1982). Health promotion: Ethical considerations. In R.B. Taylor, J.R. Vreda, & J.W. Denham (Eds.), *Health promotion: Principles and clinical applications* (pp. 393-404). Norwalk, CT: Appleton Century Crofts.

Vickerman, R.W. (1975). *The economics of leisure and recreation*. London: Macmillan.

Vickerman, R.W. (1979). *Personal and family leisure expenditure*. London: Sports Council and Social Sciences. [Research Council Joint Panel on Leisure and Recreation Research]

Volle, M., Shephard, R.J., Lavallée, H., LaBarre, R., Jéquier, J.C., & Rajic, M. (1982a). Influence of a program of required physical activity upon academic performance. In H. Lavallée & R.J. Shephard (Eds.), *Croissance et développement de l'enfant* (pp. 91-109). Trois Rivières: University of Québec at Trois Rivières, Trois Rivières, Quebec.

Volle, M., Tisal, H., LaBarre, R., Lavallée, H., Shephard, R.J., Jéquier, J.C., & Rajic, M. (1982b). Influence d'un programme expérimental d'activités physiques intégré a l'école primaire sur le développement de quelques éléments psychomoteurs. In H. Lavallée & R.J. Shephard (Eds.), *Croissance et developpement de l'enfant* (pp. 201-222). Trois Rivières: University of Québec at Trois Rivières.

Von Boerhaave, A.K. (1737). *A. Kaau. Declamatio academica de Gaudiis Alchemistarum* (p. 11). Leiden: Samuelem Luchtmans, Academie Typographum.

Waaler, H.Th., & Hjort, P.F. (1982). Physical activity, health and health economics. *Scandinavian Journal of Social Medicine Supplement*, **29**, 265-269.

Wagner, F., & Washington, V.F. (1982). Analysis of personal consumption expenditures as related to recreation, 1945-1976. *Journal of Leisure Research*, **14**, 37-46.

Walker, W.D. (1977). Changing United States life-style and declining vascular mortality: Cause or coincidence? *New England Journal of Medicine, 297*, 163-165.

Walz, F. (1978). Sport and its economic and social importance. *Olympic Review, 128*, 373-377.

Wanzel, R.S. (1974). *Determination of attitudes of employees and management of Canadian corporations toward company sponsored physical activity facilities and programs.* Doctoral dissertation, University of Alberta, Edmonton, Canada.

Wanzel, R.S. (1979). Rationale for employee fitness programs. In R.S. Wanzel (Ed.), *Employee fitness, the how to* (pp. 1-16). Toronto: Ministry of Culture and Recreation.

Ware, B. (1982). Health education in occupational settings; History has a message. *Health Education Quarterly, 9* (Suppl.), 37-41.

Watson, T. (1980). *Sociology, work and industry.* Boston: Routledge Kegan Paul.

Wear, R.F. (1983). The Campbell Soup Company program. *Preventive Medicine, 12*, 667-671.

Webster, W.D., & Reich, C.M. (1976, January/February). Benefit-cost evaluation. *Recreation Reporter.*

Wedderburn, D. (1973). The aged and society. In J.C. Brocklehurst (Ed.), *Textbook of geriatric medicine and gerontology* (pp. 692-717). Edinburgh: Churchill-Livingstone.

Weinblatt, E., Shapiro, R., Frank, C.W., & Sager, R.F. (1966). Return to work and work status following myocardial infarction. *American Journal of Public Health, 56*, 169-185.

Weinstein, M.C. (1983). Cost-effective priorities for cancer prevention. *Science, 221*, 17-23.

Weinstein, M.C., & Stason, W.B. (1977). Foundations of cost-effectiveness analysis for health and medical practices. *New England Journal of Medicine, 296*, 716-721.

Weisbrod, B.A. (1961). *Economics of public health.* Philadelphia: University of Pennsylvania Press.

Whaley, B. (1980). *Sports centre planning and provision in England and Wales.* Unpublished doctoral dissertation, University of Birmingham, Birmingham, England.

White, A.J. (1974). The inter-relationships between measures of physical fitness and measures of self-concept of selected Missouri State University male students. *Dissertation Abstract International,* **34**(8a), 4849.

Whiting, P.J., & Miller, G.M. (1977). Recreation—Tourism benefit—Measurement for policy planning. *Recreation Research Review,* **5**(1), 26-27.

Wikler, D.I. (1978). Persuasion and coercion or health: Ethical issues in government efforts to change lifestyles. *Health and Society,* **56,** 303-337.

Wilbur, C.S. (1983). The Johnson & Johnson program. *Preventive Medicine,* **12,** 672-681.

Wiley, J.A., & Camacho, T.C. (1980). Lifestyle and future health: Evidence from the Alameda County study. *Preventive Medicine,* **9,** 1-21.

Wilkins, R., & Adams, O.B. (1983). Health expectancy in Canada, late 1970s: Demographic, regional, and social dimensions. *American Journal of Public Health,* **73**(9), 1073-1080.

Wilkins, R., & Adams, O. (1983, March/April). Measuring health. *Policy Options,* pp. 28-31.

Williamson, J.W., & Van Nieuwenhuijzen, M.G. (1974). Health benefit analysis. An application to industrial absenteeism. *Journal of Occupational Medicine,* **16,** 229-233.

Willie, A.W. (1976, December). Recreation and industry. *Australian Journal of H.P.E.R.,* **74,** 20-28.

Wilman, E.A. (1980). Value of time in recreation benefit studies. *Journal of Environmental Economic Management,* **7,** 272-286.

Wilson, D.M. (1982). *Cost-effective fitness.* Vancouver, B.C.: Hydro Health Services.

Wilson, G. (1981, November 8-14). The growth business of getting fit. *The National Times* (Australia).

Wilson, L.A., & Levy, G. (1978). *Making decisions about admitting patients to a hospital department of geriatric medicine* (Abstracts). 11th International Congress of Gerontology, Tokyo.

Wolfson, A. (1974). *A health index for Ontario.* Toronto: Ministry of Treasury and Intergovernmental Affairs.

Work in America. (1973). *Report of a special task force to the U.S. Secretary of Health, Education and Welfare, prepared under the auspices of the W.E. Upjohn Institute for Employment Research.* Cambridge, MA: M.I.T. Press.

World Health Forum. (1981). Health for all by the year 2000: A Canadian perspective. *World Health Forum,* **2,** 455-461.

World Health Organization. (1948). *Official records #2*. Geneva: Author.

World Health Organization. (1980). *World health statistics annual*. Geneva: World Health Organization.

Wright, C.C. (1982). Cost-containment through health promotion programs. *Journal of Occupational Medicine*, **24**, 965-968.

Yarvote, P.M., McDonagh, T.J., Goldman, M.E., et al. (1974). Organization and evaluation of a physical fitness program in industry. *Journal of Occupational Medicine*, **16**, 589-598.

Young, J.R., & Ismail, A.H. (1976). Personality differences of adult men before and after a physical fitness program. *Research Quarterly*, **57**, 513-519.

Zohman, L.R. (1973). Early ambulation of post-myocardial infarction patients: Montefiore Hospital. In J.P. Naughton, H.K. Hellerstein, & I.C. Mohler (Eds.), *Exercise testing and exercise training in coronary heart disease* (pp. 329-336). New York: Academic Press.

Zuk, C.J., & Moore, F.D. (1980). High cost users in medical care. *New England Journal of Medicine*, **302**, 996-1002.

Index